The Newly
NON-DRINKING
Girl's Guide to
PREGNANCY

ADVICE AND SUPPORT FOR SURVIVING 40 WEEKS WITHOUT A COSMOPOLITAN

JACKIE ROSE AND
CAROLINE ANGEL, R.N., PH.D

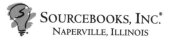

SOURCEBOOKS, INC.®
NAPERVILLE, ILLINOIS

Published by Sourcebooks, Inc.
P.O. Box 4410, Naperville, Illinois 60567–4410
(630) 961–3900
Fax: (630) 961–2168
www.sourcebooks.com

Library of Congress Cataloging-in-Publication Data

Rose, Jackie.
   The newly non-drinking girl's guide to pregnancy : advice and support
for surviving 40 weeks without a cosmopolitan / Jackie Rose and Caroline
Angel.
       p. cm.
   Includes bibliographical references and index.
   ISBN-13: 978-1-4022-0920-8 (alk. paper)
   ISBN-10: 1-4022-0920-7 (alk. paper)
   1. Pregnant women--Alcohol use. 2. Temperance. 3. Pregnancy--Popular
works. 4. Pregnant women--Social life and customs. I. Angel, Caroline.
II. Title.

HV5137.R67 2007
618.2'42--dc22

                              2007001790

      Printed and bound in the United States of America.
              VP 10 9 8 7 6 5 4 3 2 1

DEDICATION

For Dan, Abby, and Asher

—Jackie Rose

For Steve, Catherine, and Joshua

—Caroline Angel

Contents

ACKNOWLEDGMENTS

Thanks to…

Caroline Angel, for the spark and the spirit—your postpartum martini is right around the corner! Marcy Posner, for your always excellent advice, as agent and friend. Editors Bethany Brown and Shana Drehs, and the whole team at Sourcebooks, for believing in our little book and making it bigger and better. Dr. Lorne Scharf, for answering all of my questions about everything.

Our very own "Champion" Jacqueline Appleby, Safta Rachel and Dino, Zaide Shoel, Keenan, Evan, Selena, Galit, Mama + Papa, Grampy, Bubba, Dan and Darline (and your legendary breakfast spreads), Jordy, Sarah and Drew, Bubby Sandy, and Ted—for baby-sitting, support, and so much more.

The tots behind our temperance, in order of appearance: Marlo, Hunter, Abbey Bard, Liam, Ben, Madeleine, Fran, Jasper, Number Nine, Star, Matthew, Tomas, Jake, Circle, Meredith, and Amelia.

Dan my dearest, Abby my little big girl, and Asher my smasher—you're the shalom in my home…and my heart.

—*Jackie Rose*

There was so much support for the idea of this book that it gave me a jump start to getting it going.

Jackie Rose, you are my hero! Thanks for making this idea a reality—you made my dream come true! Many thanks to Marcy Posner for selling the idea and closing the deal. And many thanks to Bethany Brown, Shana Drehs, and the entire staff of Sourcebooks for your hard work and commitment to guiding our best foot forward.

I would like to thank our guest mixologists and the sources who brought them to us: Anna Getty from purestyleliving.com and her manager, Alisa Donner Hamad (Amrita) of Delight Full, Inc; Gregg Horan from Luxbar and Gibsons Restaurant in Chicago and Stephen Lombardo; and Terry Kranz from Abacus Restaurant and Ariana Hajibashi-Martin of McCrory & Associates. I would also like to thank Jennifer Stieve from the Minnesota Organization on Fetal Alcohol Syndrome, and Anne Wilson from the NJ Coalition for Prevention of Developmental Disabilities for contributing recipes from their Pregnant Pause campaigns.

Thanks to my friends and family for all your love, support, encouragement, and guidance.

Thanks, also, to my children—my daughter, Catherine, the inspiration behind this wacky idea, and Joshua.

And finally, thank you to my loving and supportive husband, Steve.

—*Caroline Angel*

FROM DRINKING FOR ONE TO EATING FOR TWO

Congratulations—you're pregnant.

Yes, you!

Don't panic.

Everything's going to be okay…

Whether the happy news comes as a complete shock or is the culmination of many years of trying to conceive, you've now officially crossed the line from Drinking for One to Eating for Two. For some of us, this is way easier said than done. (Don't worry, you can admit it; you're among friends here.) Yes, the prospect of forty long, long weeks without a single cocktail is enough to strike dread into the heart and fear into the belly of even the most moderate of imbibers.

Happily, there are also many joys of expectant motherhood. If you're interested in hearing about them, however, this book is not for you. Suffice it to say that we, too, salute you on your luminous complexion and general gestational glowingness and greatness. First flutters, belly bumps, baby showers…it's all so darn wonderful. And oh, when you see your baby's face for the first time? Yeah, you'll fall in love. (Or not. For some people, that comes later.)

Can we move on now?

Good.

So while there are many joys associated with having a bun baking in the oven, giving up alcohol is definitely not one of them. It's annoying enough that pregnancy can make us feel, on occasion, hideously deformed, vomity, varicose-veiny, morbidly obese, farty, and moody…and now we're expected to give up our Cosmo, colada, or glass of wine, too? Personally, we find this to be far more frightening than hemorrhoids or stretch marks, which, odds are, you are also about to experience in all their glory. But that's another story altogether.

Where were we? Ah, yes. Back to the booze, then. Without a little something to calm our nerves, how are we supposed to relax under the weight of the world, not to mention under the burden of our ever-expanding bellies? It's not like our jobs are getting any easier—they're still stressful, require long hours, and hijack virtually all our mental energy—and now we have to get through them without the pleasure of knowing that the day's end brings a double martini or half a bottle of our favorite Chardonnay. Why, it's positively alarming.

More terrifying still—what about all those business dinners? How can anyone be expected to endure a three-hour borefest with elderly clients sans Syrah? Equally awful, a working liquid lunch with the boss, minus the liquid, is about as much fun as a Brazilian bikini wax—and nearly as hairy. (Unless, of course, you are the boss, in which case we respect you greatly and very much enjoy working with you.)

And if you think your professional life is challenging without alcohol, wait until you experience your best friend's three-day bachelorette party blowout in Vegas *without a single sip.*

Forty Weeks and Counting...

If this is your first, you're probably a little unsure of what to expect. Your body's poised to undergo many months of serious readjusting, to say nothing of the storm brewing between your ears. Sore nipples, swollen belly, huge boobs (boobs that may seem even *bigger* than your belly, in fact)...then there's the labor, delivery, stitches, bleeding...diapers, feeding, crying, sleeping (yes, we're talking about you *and* the baby, here)...postpartum depression, aggression, repression...sex, love, joy, pain, diets, career, religion, existentialism, fashion...and that's really just a small sampling of what'll be going on over at your house for the next twelve months or so.

You're teetering on the brink of a new life, a strange new world where what *you* want not only doesn't matter, but where even your most basic needs and desires—at least for a little while—will actually cease to exist. Motherhood is bearing down on you like a freight train. Your mind is spinning with questions and concerns and hopes and dreams.

If you've already had a kid, at least you know that it *is* worth it. Still, you're heading back to the starting gate again. Your new baby, we can assure you, will have complete disregard for everything you think you know about pregnancy, childbirth, and motherhood. Your mind is spinning with questions and concerns and hopes and dreams.

Sounds like a pretty good time for a martini, doesn't it?

The sad irony is that you're absolutely right. With all that's going on in your life these days, you deserve a drink now more than ever. Hopefully, you already have an inkling as to why that's not such a good idea. If not, we'll set you straight.

No need to be afraid. We aren't the preachy type, and our goal here is not to chastise or humiliate anybody for being perfectly human. In fact, we've survived four dry and grueling gestations between the two of us, so we wholeheartedly commiserate with your sudden pregnancy-induced sobriety. Yes, we know all about those missed Bloody Marys over Sunday brunch, the margarita-free summers, the soft cider Thanksgivings, the ginger ale toasts on New Year's Eve, and, worst of all, the empty champagne glasses on Valentine's Day (though you should do pretty well in the chocolate department this year).

The reason we're the perfect ones to guide you through this bittersweet rite of parental passage is because we love our liquor as much as the next gal, and know better than anyone how hard it can be to put all that aside for the sake of some unborn stranger roughly the size of a sesame seed. But between us, over time, we somehow stumbled upon a way that works—a system that involves embracing new oral fixations and relaxation techniques along with adopting a sort of "be prepared" approach to alcohol and all its social, mental, and physical implications. One by one, we conquered every demon that came our way, and we wrote this guide in the hopes that our experiences will help you to do the same.

Your First Act of Mommyhood

It's true for many "moderate" drinkers—whom, for our purposes, we'll define as those of us who enjoy a cocktail (or two) most weeknights and, ahem, maybe a few more on the occasional Friday or Saturday evening—that giving up alcohol for your unborn child will constitute a major life event. But as the first step in the process of becoming a good parent, it is an absolute must.

Your number-one job as a mom-to-be is to provide as safe and as nurturing an environment as possible. From this point on, what you want is irrelevant; what your kid *needs* is imperative. There's more room to wiggle on this once the baby's actually born. For now, though, you exist only as an incubator. Sorry, dear. It comes with the job.

Unlike grande mocha lattes, spicy tuna rolls, Diet Pepsi, and acrylic tips, alcohol does not fall into that hazy Should-I-or-Shouldn't-I? category of indulgences we wrestle with during our gestations. While most obstetricians and midwives will tell you that moderation is key when it comes to caffeine or those evil, nitrate-soaked luncheon meats, we've never heard of a single one who'd condone alcohol as an acceptable form of fetal nourishment. If yours does, you may want to rethink your choice.

We won't elaborate just yet on all the negative effects of drinking during pregnancy, or why even a little isn't a good idea. Suffice it to say that medical researchers have been unable to pinpoint exactly how much or how little alcohol it takes to have a detrimental impact on a baby in utero, and that the effects of excessive drinking in its worst form—Fetal Alcohol Syndrome (FAS)—can mean a lifetime of mental, physical, and social consequences for your little one.

Scared yet?

You should be, because this is serious stuff. The good news is that these health problems are 100 percent avoidable. Your desire to be the best mother you can be, even at this early stage, is what will give you the strength to carry on through the next nine months as sober as a judge.

See? Even before the baby arrives, you're already a great mom—you're making some changes, doing the right thing. That kid in there is lucky to have you!

Yeah, we know…it still kinda sucks. And unless you had the foresight to give up drinking entirely before you got knocked up, you're stuck with cold turkey. Some people find it helpful to think of alcohol abstinence as very good practice for what lies ahead—putting your kids' needs above your own for as long as you both shall live. (And you thought your wedding vows were tough!) So go to the freezer, get that bottle of vodka, and pour it down the drain. If your significant other has the audacity to complain, simply explain to him that as a show of solidarity for your selfless teetotalism, the very least he can do is stand by your side—as long as he's in your presence—and that if he refuses, the empty bottles will be summarily smashed over his head.

Keep pouring…

Keep pouring…

That's it!

Now smile—there are plenty of other ways to catch a buzz, relieve tension, and celebrate life.

The Tools of Teetotalism

We're here not only to help you negotiate the oft-tricky task of abstaining through the next nine months and possibly beyond, but also to guide you as delicately as possible through the minefield of alcohol-related situations you're bound to encounter along the way.

First things first. What exactly are the issues surrounding drinking and gestating, anyway? We'll answer all your questions, from what happens if you drank like a fish *before* you peed on that stick (don't worry too much—we'll try to put your mind at ease, once and for all) to something we'd been wondering for a long time: if it's okay for French women to guzzle wine during *their* pregnancies, why can't we?

Many of the pregnant women we know (including us) were most troubled by alcohol-related issues that arose during the first trimester. Giving up happy hour, for example—not at *all* fun. And if, for whatever reason, you're not ready to share the good news just yet, keeping it quiet when your sudden sobriety is raising eyebrows is bound to be a challenge. At work, the timing of your big announcement may be particularly sensitive in some situations, say, if you were recently hired, or if there's been a rash of maternity leave lately. Nervous superiors have probably been monitoring your waistline since your wedding, and to them, your giving up alcohol is a sure sign of impending doom. Friends and family, too, may need to be subtly distracted from the change in your drinking habits. Don't feel bad, guilty, or deceptive about it, either: your right to privacy in matters of pregnancy is always paramount.

Fear not: we've got lots of ways for you to dodge prying or personal questions about why you're suddenly tossing back cranberry juice at the Christmas party, when last year you won the eggnog-drinking contest. Knowing a few simple tactics and diversion techniques is really all it takes to secure your secret for as long as you like.

Right now, the most important thing for you to keep in mind is that there *are* ways to simulate the mental, physical, and social benefits of a cocktail or two without drinking a single drop. We'll show you how to create a new happy hour in your home, ditching the alcohol while retaining the relaxing effects of this essential after-work ritual. To keep the spirit alive, fifty teetotally terrific mocktail recipes are scattered throughout the pages of this book. If you're still looking for a buzz, we'll also reveal our Four Favorite Fetus-Friendly Ways to catch one. And yes, sex and chocolate are on the list.

Of course, just because you've got baby on board doesn't mean you have to be a shut-in for the next nine months. But what about those sticky situations that just wouldn't feel right without a drink in your hand? Barbecues, bachelorette parties, birthdays, bar mitzvahs, weddings, wakes…all can still be experienced to the fullest. And if bar-hopping was formerly your top source of aerobic and social activity, no need to give it up—provided you negotiate this tricky territory with your burgeoning belly in mind.

Nevertheless, we acknowledge that forty-plus weeks of abstinence from alcohol isn't exactly going to be a breeze for every Newly Non-Drinking Girl. So for anyone out there who feels like she might be in need of a little bit of extra help, we've also come up with our very own sobriety system—Twelve Sober Steps for Nine Long Months, designed just for expectant moms—along with an exhaustive rundown of the professional help, recovery programs, and support networks available.

The time will soon come when the key to the minibar will be yours again. After the baby's born, you may choose to indulge in a little nip now and then to help take the edge off the loneliness and stress—umm, we mean, to help *celebrate* the many delightful joys and blessings of motherhood, which you'll shortly be experiencing in all their glory and wonder. In fact, the postpartum period presents a slew of new questions and concerns all its own, especially if you choose to breast-feed. We'll cover them all.

You Can Do It!

Still not convinced?

Over the next fifty or sixty years, you will no doubt encounter plenty of suitable occasions in which motherhood calls for a nice, stiff drink. We promise. The day your five-year-old starts kindergarten, maybe, or while you wait in the dark for your newly-licensed sixteen-year-old to pull into the driveway two hours past curfew. Parenthood, by its very nature, is fraught with sadness and joy, anxiety and relief, madness and sanity—sometimes all at once. There will be broken bones, broken hearts, birthdays, graduations, engagements, weddings, births, hirings, firings, promotions, divorces, anniversaries, retirements—and through it all, you'll be pretty much free to celebrate or unwind as you see fit. But for now, sister, you're stuck.

Remember when we said we'd leave the mushy stuff to someone else? Well, we lied. Whether you realize this yet or not, the moment you deliver your baby, an amazing thing happens…something almost as frightening as it is wonderful: a little piece of your heart will also be leaving your body that day and will begin beating outside of it. And no matter how old she gets or how far he travels, your child will forever remain in possession of it, for as long as you are alive. Never will you love anyone like you love your kids. Not your parents, not your spouse, not even yourself.

So let's try this again, shall we?

Congratulations—you're pregnant.

Yes, you!

Don't panic.

Everything's going to be okay…

And you're going to do it all without a single drop of alcohol.

Yeah, you heard us—*not one drop.*

Here's how.

Fifty Virgin Drinks for Forty Vexing Weeks

In the spirit of spiritless sisterhood, we're here to offer you fifty virgin drinks for those forty vexing weeks. Although we have quite a range of experience in the drink-mixing department—from playing bartender at home to years of taste-testing on the seedy nightclub scene—we cannot claim to have created *all* these fantastic recipes ourselves. While some are original formulations, others are classics you may already be familiar with, since in the world of alcohol-free drinks, there are certain gold standards—tried-and-true recipes, just like that close-to-your-heart Cosmo or classic screwdriver—whose formulations should not be messed with.

If you feel like getting creative with concoctions on your own, we recommend you visit websites like drinksmixer.com or idrink.com, which were not only important sources of inspiration for us, but which also encourage all you amateur mixologists out there to submit your recipes to share with the masses. Equally appreciated are our guest mixologists—Anna Getty of purestyleliving.com, Terry Kranz of Abacus restaurant in Dallas, Gregg Horan of Gibsons and Luxbar in Chicago, and Pregnant Pause campaigns from New Jersey and Minnesota—who generously contributed several outstanding original mocktails for these pages.

And now, a few notes on usage for *The Newly Non-Drinking Girl's Guide to Pregnancy:*

- Remember that employing the right barware is crucial when trying to convince yourself you're feeling a little tipsy, and it also conveys a certain measure of respect for the drink itself. (Try drinking a Maternitini out of a sippy cup and you'll see what we mean.)
- We highly recommend that you invest in a blender, since we found that a number of the better mocktail recipes out there need to whipped, frappéd, and/or frozen into fabulousness.
- To achieve the desired effect in frozen drinks, shaved ice is best. (We don't know why, exactly; it just blends better.) Buy a bag of store-made ice, 7-Eleven-style, to keep on hand.
- Invest in a selection of flavored syrups at the beginning of your pregnancy. You'll be glad they're there when you need them.

- Please vary the ingredients to suit your specific tastes and preferences. A little more cranberry or a little less tonic may be the difference between bland and mind-blowing.
- Finally, for relevancy's sake, we placed each of our fifty recipes in the chapter that seemed to suit it best, but feel free to whip 'em up whenever and wherever you like—the one exception being Number 50, the Baby Bottle Cosmo (you'll see why when you get there). In the meantime, we hope you enjoy each and every one of these liquor-free libations as much as we have.

We wish you all a safe and healthy pregnancy!

FREQUENTLY FEARED QUESTIONS:

Debunking the Myths, Defining the Medicine

"What happens in Vegas, stays in Vegas, right?!"
—*Riana L., 27, Miami, FL*

Now that you've excitedly welcomed/grudgingly accepted the good news, let's move on to some business. Here's where you'll find the answers to any questions you may have—including all the medical issues, facts, and myths—about drinking and gestating. While we've tried to consider every, um, *conceivable* situation that may currently be worrying, puzzling, or mortifying you, it's by no means an exhaustive list. So, if you're left wondering what to do if you accidentally get pushed into a vat of beer, ask your doctor or midwife.

Let's get some business out of the way first. Please be assured that we're here to help put your mind at ease, but we're also going to tell it to you like it is. Since this is a pretty serious subject, you may not like the answers to some of the questions. That's okay, because no matter what happened in Vegas, the best thing you can do *from this point on*—for both your conscience and your developing baby—is to stop drinking right away.

Now, now.

Take a deep breath.

Try and stay calm.

Remember that there is a huge difference between alcohol *use* and alcohol *abuse*. The negative effects a mother's drinking might have on her fetus are generally associated with alcohol abuse—that is, repeated and prolonged exposure to alcohol. That's why those few drinks you had before you found out you were pregnant—or, let's be honest here, the ones you may have had *after* you already knew, but weren't fully aware of the possible consequences—are *not* the end of the world. But more on this subject later.

For now, as we've said, be aware that it is not known exactly how much alcohol it takes to hurt an unborn baby or what the so-called thresholds are for negative outcomes. Which is why, for the purposes of answering the questions below and because it is the very premise upon which this little book is based, we're promoting a zero-tolerance policy when it comes to pregnancy and alcohol. Drinking and gestating, like drinking and driving, is a lot like playing Russian roulette with your kid's life.

Ready to continue?

Good.

Because chances are whatever happened in Vegas *will* stay in Vegas, never to be thought of again, or relegated to that category of regrets to be looked back upon fondly from the safe haven of No Damage Done. Unless, of course, Sin City is where you got knocked up in the first place. In that case, what happened in Vegas will most definitely *not* be staying in Vegas. Rather, it will be coming home with you on the plane, then hijacking your body, mind, and soul for the next nine months and far, far beyond.

But don't worry about any of that just yet. There are plenty more pressing things to think about between now and then.

If all else fails, you can always kick it out when it turns eighteen anyway.

Each one of the drinks in this chapter contains an antidote for some sort of pregnancy-induced pain-in-the-belly. The last thing you need with all those crazy questions swirling around in your head is the distraction and discomfort of nausea and bloating. So here's to relief—for both your body and your mind.

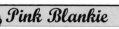

Pink Blankie

(aka Watermelon Aqua Fresca)

If you're thinking pink, this one's for you—a delicious, refreshing, and baby-shower friendly recipe, with a main ingredient well-known for fighting nausea! (It may be the sugary water content in the fruit that does it.) Just try not to eat all the watermelon while you're preparing the recipe, or there'll be none left for anyone else.

Ice

½ large watermelon (about 3 pounds)

2 cups sparkling water, plus more if needed

Pinch salt (optional)

1 or 2 tbsp. lime juice (optional)

Save yourself some time and buy a seedless watermelon. You can pick out the white seeds if they bug you, but we wouldn't bother (remember, this is supposed to be fun). Using your fancy little melon baller (this is what that bridal shower gift was intended for), scoop watermelon into little balls or, if you're not fancy schmancy, slice into little cubes with a knife.

Place the watermelon in a blender with 2 cups of sparkling water. If salty is your thing, add a pinch. Blend until the mixture is smooth, then strain into a pitcher. Add lime juice to taste. Serve on the rocks in a margarita glass. Garnish with a lime wedge.

Quick Answers to All Your Quaffing Questions

Q: *"If I drink, will my baby get drunk too?"*

Yes!

The simple truth is, once alcohol hits your stomach, it enters your bloodstream quickly and easily. (That's the fun of it, right?) Your boozy blood then makes a beeline for that little person you're charged with protecting via the placenta—an extraordinary pizza-shaped organ that, during pregnancy, delivers nutrients and oxygen directly to your baby and helps it expel waste. It all makes for an awfully alcoholic amniotic marinade—one your baby will be stewing in for quite some time. Secondhand intoxication, therefore, is not only possible, it's virtually guaranteed. Not really an ideal environment for junior, especially since she's still years away from being able to walk a straight line to begin with.

Q: *"Be honest—what are the actual effects of alcohol abuse during pregnancy? Aren't they being overstated by the media and medical communities in this age of political correctness?"*

Nobody's exaggerating anything. According to the American College of Obstetricians and Gynecologists, which likes to form its opinions on a little something called the scientific method, there are four major outcomes of prenatal alcohol abuse: spontaneous abortion, birth defects, central nervous system impairment, and Fetal

Alcohol Syndrome. Other problems, such as intrauterine growth retardation, preterm labor, delivery complications, low birth weight, and even stillbirth have been reported.

These complications appear to be linked to *moderate to heavy alcohol use* during pregnancy—that is to say, little empirical evidence actually exists to suggest that light drinking before you found out (or even later) is capable of causing the devastating effects seen in the children of heavy drinkers. In this day and age, however, most North Americans—and the health organizations, media outlets, legal communities, social bodies, and commercial enterprises of which we form a part—tend to err on the side of caution when it comes to such things. Ask the California Raisin Company if its products are safe to consume during pregnancy and the answer won't be too far off the one you'd get from a drug manufacturer: "We don't know for sure. No conclusive studies have been done. Consult your doctor first."

It's not only because we're anal, overly politically correct, or even fearful of litigation—though this may very well be true—but also because we're pragmatists. We like to cover our bases, especially when it comes to the health and well-being of our most precious commodity—our kids. Since a threshold for safe alcohol consumption during pregnancy has yet to be pinpointed, and the research on the subject seems to be changing almost daily, the evils of prenatal boozing will continue to be expounded by everyone with a soapbox to stand on.

So, while we'd love to tell you a drink here and there during your pregnancy is fine and will likely have no ill effects on your kid, we can't—even though it's probably true. We have a responsibility to take the high road, just like you do.

Q: *"What exactly is Fetal Alcohol Syndrome?"*

Fetal Alcohol Syndrome (FAS) is the most serious of the so-called Fetal Alcohol Spectrum Disorders (FASD), an all-encompassing term used to designate the wide array of physical, developmental, and emotional problems resulting from a baby's exposure to alcohol in utero. Kids with FAS have a set of distinguishing physical characteristics (facial abnormalities, skeletal deformities, eye and ear problems, small brains, and heart and organ malformations), cognitive disabilities (mental retardation, developmental and motor delays, and language and learning disorders), and behavioral problems (hyperactivity, ADHD, and poor judgment, reasoning, socialization, and impulse control), among others. The effects of FAS are unfortunately irreversible, though symptoms can be managed through medical, educational, and therapeutical intervention.

According to the March of Dimes—the world's leading nonprofit organization dedicated to the research and prevention of birth defects and infant mortality—FAS is the leading known cause of mental retardation. Estimates suggest that in the United States, roughly 10,000 kids born each year have FAS, making it more prevalent than spina bifida, Down syndrome, muscular dystrophy, and HIV *combined*. Because of this, FAS is an extremely serious public health problem. And since it's also entirely preventable, the importance of public awareness and education cannot be overstated.

Q: *"Should I just be worried about FAS, or are there other less serious risks associated with drinking during pregnancy?"*

In order to confirm a diagnosis of FAS, a very specific set of criteria must be met. Around three times the amount of kids born with FAS are actually diagnosed with Partial Fetal Alcohol Syndrome (PFAS) or Fetal Alcohol Effects (FAE) instead, meaning they show some of the symptoms of FAS, but not all. Cases of PFAS can range from the very mild, displaying just one or two symptoms, to the very severe, involving a complicated array of disorders similar to full-blown FAS.

Absent an FAS, PFAS, or FAE diagnosis, affected babies are generally divided into two categories: those with Alcohol-Related Birth Defects (ARBD), involving physical aspects such as heart and eye abnormalities, and those with Alcohol-Related Neurodevelopmental Disorder (ARND), distinguished by cognitive and behavioral issues. In all, Fetal Alcohol Spectrum disorders affect 40,000 infants every single year, and possibly even more, due to suspected underreporting. Unlike FAS, which is the result of heavy alcohol consumption during pregnancy, ARBD and ARND have been know to occur in the children of light to moderate drinkers, which is why it's absolutely crucial to *stop drinking completely* the moment you find out you're pregnant.

Bugs Bunny Special

Yeah, we know, it's orange. But so what if it looks a little weird? It's super healthy and perfect for getting back on track on those mornings-after-a-chocolate-binge. The vitamin B6, abundant in carrots, is also known to help quell morning sickness. Baby bonus: moms who drink carrot juice during their pregnancies are apparently more likely to have kids who like their first carrots.

Ice (optional)

3 oz. carrot juice

3 oz. apple juice

For convenience, use store–bought juices. Mix portions together in equal parts and serve in a highball glass, on ice if you prefer. Garnish with a carrot stick greens, and everything. That's all, folks!

Q: *"Now I'm completely terrified—I didn't know I was pregnant and I had a few drinks. What have I done?"*

Chances are, nothing.

Those of you who were prescient (or lucky) enough to be avoiding alcohol altogether while trying to get pregnant can knock this worry off your ever-growing list of concerns and get back to obsessing over items like swollen ankles and the debate over sushi. If you *weren't* trying to get knocked up—or if you miscalculated your dates, have irregular periods, or the dog ate your calendar—read on.

Along with queries about over-the-counter cold and flu medications and painkillers, this is probably the number-one question fielded by obstetricians and midwives after "What's my due date?" Most health care professionals will quickly put your mind at ease—one Corona on a hot summer day or that short snifter of brandy you indulged in to help you catch your z's is really nothing to lose sleep over.

Biology has ensured that your beloved little cluster of cells, though fragile, is also able to weather many of the storms ahead. Morning sickness, for example, which often starts around week six and for some women lasts until week 1,132 (college graduation), can prove to be a serious obstacle to adequate nutritional intake. But somehow, even if all you can force down are grape es and soda crackers, your baby's bones and brain ~~~ ~~~rt continue to form properly and at the correct rate. Similarly, the alcohol contained in a few Mai Tais is unlikely to exact serious damage.

Here's how it works in a nutshell: alcohol intake during any stage of pregnancy, especially early on, is known to have a teratogenic effect on the fetus, meaning it's capable of causing birth defects. During the first trimester, it not only kills already-existing brain cells, but prevents new ones from forming, and causes other physical abnormalities, too. The thing with alcohol, though, as you probably have memorized by now, is that nobody's been able to pinpoint exactly how much of it and when, over the course of a pregnancy, is enough to cause harm. Even the same level of exposure affects different babies in different ways. (It's a point we will probably continue to hammer home until everybody out there understands why this potentially problematic uncertainty is reason enough to promote a zero-tolerance approach to alcohol during pregnancy.) In general, however, the more alcohol a pregnant woman consumes and the more often she drinks it is directly related to the severity of the outcome.

That's the bad news.

The good news is what we *do* know for sure: FAS and other serious problems are caused by heavy drinking— we're talking four to five drinks a day here, and that's day after day after day. That's not what you did, so there's no reason to drive yourself crazy.

Yes, legions of fertile, hooch-loving mamas have trod this path smooth before you, to no ill effect. Their ten-fingered, ten-toed offspring generally do just as well on their SATs as those whose teetotaling mothers sealed themselves in plastic bubble wrap for the duration of their gestations. Though nothing is ever guaranteed until you're holding that healthy, screeching kid in your arms, there's virtually no evidence to suggest that a couple of drinks drunk early on is likely to do irreversible harm.

Q: *"So, is there a safer time to drink during pregnancy?"*

No time is the right time. While some studies suggest that drinking earlier in pregnancy is worse—as little as one or two drinks a day throughout the first trimester may be associated with a higher risk of birth defects—alcohol consumption during the last two trimesters has been known to increase the chance of miscarriage and premature labor or delivery, interfere with brain growth, impair central nervous system development, and cause inadequate weight gain in the baby, among other things.

First things first. If you're trying to get pregnant, it's a good idea to avoid the hooch altogether, or at the very least save it for the preovulatory phase of your menstrual cycle. (Indeed, the aphrodisiac effects of a good, um, stiff drink have certainly resulted in more healthy, normal babies than could possibly be counted.) If, however, you imbibed in the two-week window between conception and when that thin pink line appeared on the home pregnancy test (HPT), fear not—the alcohol contained in a measly drink or two is highly unlikely to have any effect on your zipping zygote or burgeoning blastocyst.

A final word of warning: just because this happens to be true, we in no way mean to suggest that it's okay to sneak a drink now and then. As we've said before, different pregnancies are affected by alcohol in different ways. The precise thresholds of safe consumption are not known—its effects on the fetus on a week-by-week basis remain a mystery. So as soon as you know you're pregnant, the bar is closed!

Q: *"My sister's getting married. Can't I have even ONE glass of champagne at her wedding?"*

Some people may tell you that it's bad luck not to partake during the toast to the bride at a wedding, our zero-tolerance rule notwithstanding. If you really feel you must, wet your lips out of someone else's glass. That way, you won't be tempted to overindulge. Also keep in mind that if you're not showing yet, judgmental glares and wagging fingers won't be a deterring factor, so you'll have to find strength from within. If you are showing, expect a few shocked looks or maybe even a comment or two if anyone sees you taking a sip.

Two by Anna Getty

When we went looking for some expertise in the area of holistic health, we turned to our friend, Anna Getty, the LA-based prenatal yoga specialist and instructor for the popular *Divine Mother Prenatal Yoga Series* DVD. She recommends ginger-based drinks to ward off morning sickness. We couldn't agree more.

The Stork and Mommy

This delightful beverage takes its shape and form from *The Dark and Stormy.* Speaking of your moods, there may be a few dark and stormies passing through your place over the next few months as those pregnancy hormones take over your body and your mind.

Ice

2 tsp. dark cherry syrup or black currant syrup (to replace the dark rum—boo hoo)

6–8 oz. ginger beer

First, pour syrup into bottom of a collins glass. Add ice, then pour in ginger beer. Stir well. Enjoy!

The Mama-To-Be Tummy Tamer

This warm and soothing tea can be a lifesaver as bouts of nausea rear their ugly heads. Don't worry, for this too shall pass. We like to enjoy a cup with a good book.

1 inch fresh ginger, peeled and finely sliced*

2–3 sprigs fresh mint*

16 oz. water

Honey to sweeten

Place all ingredients (except honey) into a pot and bring to a boil. Simmer for twenty minutes. Strain hot liquid into a mug. Add honey to taste. Makes two servings, or simply double the recipe and store in the fridge for a quick tummy–saver.

Variation: You can also add some soy milk or regular milk to make it creamy.

* If you're unable to find the fresh ingredients or don't have any on hand, take one bag of ginger tea and one bag of mint tea and place them in a pot with 16 oz. of water. Bring the bags to a boil, then simmer for five minutes.

Q: *"That's all well and good for the lightweight, but I didn't know I was pregnant and one night I went out with my friends and I drank...A LOT! What have I done?"*

Again, chances are, nothing.

About half of all pregnancies in the U.S. are

unplanned, but even if you *were* trying, we know that just because you have babies on the brain doesn't mean life doesn't get in the way sometimes. Celebrating, mourning, and plain old bad judgment happen to the best of us, as suggested by the following quotes from real live drinking girls who hit the bottle hard before they knew:

"I must have had twenty piña coladas on our honeymoon cruise…we found out I was pregnant three weeks later."

—Jasmine P., 32, Des Moines, IA

"My friend left her husband, so we went out to celebrate with three bottles of champagne. A few months later, I thought I was in early menopause, but guess what? I was already halfway through my second trimester!"

—Charlotte C., 44, Burlington, VT

"The day I passed the New York bar exam, I drank five shots of tequila—and that was just before dinner…"

—Christine W., 24, New York, NY

"Our doctor told us we'd never conceive without help (I have polycystic ovarian syndrome *and* my husband has low sperm motility). We decided to go for one last hurrah in the Napa Valley before starting our first round of IVF. My weeklong hangover after we came home turned out to be morning sickness!"

—*Marina S., 38, Denver, CO*

Despite nearly driving themselves insane with worry, all these women—and countless others in similar situations—went on to deliver healthy, normal babies.

Binge drinking is classically defined as having five or more drinks on a single occasion. We know—that's a lot less than you'd think, right? Well, don't freak out. According to the March of Dimes, pregnant alcoholics and chronic binge drinkers go on to have babies with FAS only about 6 percent of the time. (A statistically significant number, of course, but one which may help put your own dalliance with alcohol into perspective.)

Still, you should definitely tell your doctor or midwife that you misbehaved, since he or she will likely help alleviate your fears rather than compound them. As your pregnancy progresses, your health care practitioner will want to follow your baby carefully, exactly as he or she would with those patients who didn't end up dancing on the table at their fifteen-year high school reunion with a lampshade on their head.

So now that you know you're pregnant, and you're providing baby with a nice, comfy, alcohol-free womb of her own, give yourself a break and stop worrying. It's the best thing you can do for both your own sanity and that blessed little bun rising in your oven.

Chunky Monkey

Not too original. Not too chic. But this one's so good and so simple to make that we just had to include it. By the way, the potassium in bananas helps control pregnancy-related swelling and leg cramps.

1 frozen, very ripe banana (freeze in advance)

8 oz. 2% milk

Chocolate syrup, to taste

Start by blending the banana and milk until smooth, then slowly add the chocolate syrup directly into the blender, mixing between squirts of chocolate syrup. When your chocolate saturation point has been met, pour into a colada glass. Garnish with an umbrella for kicks.

Q: *"Come on—pregnant women in France drink wine all the time! Why can't I?"*

If all the pregnant women in France jumped off the Eiffel Tower, would you? Different cultures have different ideas when it comes to alcohol and pregnancy and drinking in general. But you live here, and as w discussed earlier, North America is home to a dazzling array of gestational and recreational prohibitions, for pragmatism's sake. So while Henri and Marie might taste their first hot toddies straight from the sippy cup, Henry and Mary will have to wait 'til they turn twenty-one.

Again, it's all about not taking any chances. Just because your mom didn't strap you into a car seat thirty years ago and you turned out fine doesn't mean you'd let your kid go beltless these days, does it? For some babies, swapping red wine with amniotic fluid might lead to no detrimental effects, while for others, a nightly post-prandial *digestif* might be enough to cause permanent damage. Until we know exactly how much—or rather, how little—alcohol it takes to harm babies in bellies, *laissez faire.* Why risk it?

Q: *"But my doctor said an occasional drink is okay. Why should I believe you?"*

Doctors and midwives, like the rest of us, are human beings. They are not all teetotaling puritans, nor are they all up-to-date on every single study published on the topic of alcohol and pregnancy. Many will tell you not to drink, but add a little nudge-nudge-wink-wink, one-won't-kill-you qualifier. Why shouldn't you believe this individual, whom you've entrusted with the care and delivery of your precious cargo—especially when the office Christmas party is just around the corner?

One recent study suggests that many health care providers might need a little refresher course when it comes pre-baby boozing. In a self-administered questionnaire returned by six hundred American College of Obstetricians and Gynecologists (ACOG) members, only 22 percent think that total abstinence is the best way to avoid all the major adverse outcomes of drinking during pregnancy, many weren't sure how many drinks it takes to do harm, and *a full 6 percent* believe eight or more drinks a week or five or more drinks on a single occasion to be fine, despite the College's zero-tolerance stance on drinking and pregnancy. The ACOG's conclusion? It needs to do more to make sure doctors push prohibition to their pregnant patients. Until then, it's up to you to use your best judgment—no matter who's telling you otherwise.

Q: *"I heard wine and beer are safer than hard alcohol. Is this true?"*

Short answer? You wish.

Long answer? Like so-called "light" cigarettes, wine and beer do contain That Which Is Forbidden during pregnancy. We're not going to lie to you, though: wine and beer have less alcohol than spirits, which also means that people tend to drink more of them to achieve the same effect. Beer, lager, and ale generally come in at between 4 and 8 percent alcohol by volume (ABV); wine, at 10 to 15 percent ABV. Most spirits, whose strength is measured by "proof"—twice the percentage of alcohol by volume; a bottle of 100-proof whiskey therefore contains 50 percent alcohol—pack a serious punch. Wine and beer, therefore, may seem safer by comparison, but don't be deceived. Wine, beer, brandy, gin, peach schnapps, malt liquor…they all contain alcohol, no matter what the proof or ABV, so the best idea is to steer clear of even mildly alcoholic beverages altogether. Remember, the idea here is to wean yourself of the stuff completely, not just minimize the damage.

Q: *"So I'll just stick with nonalcoholic beer and wine, right?"*

Did you know that many women report a strong craving for beer during pregnancy—even those who normally despise the stuff? You might also be surprised to learn that nonalcoholic beer and wine contains—surprise!— alcohol. By law, any beverage with 0.5 percent ABV or less can be classified as nonalcoholic. So you could, at least in theory, get drunk on nonalcoholic beer (although you'd run out of toilet paper or explode well before you made it that far). It's also possible that fake beer and wine could increase any cravings you may be having for the real thing, which is why we recommend sticking to root beer and pickles at all times. Frankly, we find the fake stuff tastes like slop anyway. And wouldn't you rather have a marvelous mocktail than a bad excuse for a beer?

Mother Earth

Avocados are an amazing source of folic acid, which you are certainly buffing up on these days. For the record, we never thought the recipe below would taste any good, either. Boy, were we wrong...

$\frac{1}{2}$ cup ice

$\frac{1}{2}$ an avocado (not too ripe)

1 $\frac{1}{2}$ cups milk

Up to 3 tbsp. sugar

Blend ice, avocado, and milk for a minute or so. Then slowly add in sugar, tasting as you go to avoid "sickeningly sweet." Pour into a highball glass. Enjoy.

Q: *"But what about alcohol as an ingredient in food?"*

Fear not—you won't have to give up that divine port-wine reduction smothering the veal scallopini at your favorite bistro. Same thing goes for the Rum-n-Raisin ice cream and penne alla vodka. That's because most of the alcohol these foods contain is burned off during the cooking process, leaving nothing but a rich, boozy after-taste that complements the flavor of so many of our favorite dishes. There's hardly enough hard stuff in any of it to get you even remotely intoxicated, unless you count the sugar rush. So when it comes to food, just use common sense. Enjoying the coq-au-vin at Chez Panisse is fine (in fact, we highly recommend it). Scarfing down three boxes of liquor-soaked chocolate-covered cherries? Not so much.

Q: *"My favorite facial toner contains alcohol. Do I have to give it up?"*

Just don't drink it. Alcohol (not the tasty kind) is an ingredient in tons of beauty products, from sunscreens and face creams to hair sprays and nail polishes. On a sidenote, alcohol has a drying effect, so it actually makes for a decent weapon in your war against the oily break-outs your raging hormones have in store for you, provided your skin isn't too sensitive to its effects.

Q: *"What about, you know, 'internal' products?"*

Even products containing alcohol that are designed to be put *in* your mouth—such as mouthwash and toothpaste—are fine during pregnancy, as long as you don't actually ingest any of the stuff in large quantities. (If you still prefer your oral hygiene products be of the virgin variety, there are several alcohol-free brands on the market; just check the labels.) As for those over-the-counter cough syrups—well-known as intoxicants to legions of high schoolers around the globe due to their buzz-inducing ingredients like alcohol and dextromethorphan—women should always consult their doctors before use, since some kinds are known to be safer during pregnancy than others.

*Ooh...*you meant douches? Avoid them for now, not because they contain small amounts of alcohol, but because douching during pregnancy has been linked to an increased risk of ectopic pregnancy, life-threatening air embolisms, preterm delivery, and bacterial vaginosis. Oh...you meant enemas? Avoid any that contain alcohol, and ask your doctor about the rest. Ancient Romans and rowdy frat boys have been known to get drunk fast by administering alcohol enemas to each other, since the colon absorbs alcohol and releases it into the bloodstream much quicker than the stomach can. So while constipation is a real bummer, there are other solutions besides enemas. We know—you were just asking for a friend.

Blue Belly Shake

Just a variant on a familiar fruit, milk, and blender theme here. But the blueberries are powerful antioxidants, full of fiber, a good source of folic acid, and may even help prevent urinary tract infections (big bonus!).

½ cup ice

8 oz. milk

4 oz. blueberries

Up to 1 tbsp. sugar

Break out the blender. Best to blend the milk and berries first, then add the sugar to taste. Serve in a collins or highball glass, and garnish with fresh blueberries.

Q: *"Alcoholism runs in my family. Will I be passing on some sort of drunk gene to my baby?"*

In 2004, researchers identified a gene linked to alcoholism. Even if you did have the wonky wiring in question (which you'd have no way of knowing, by the way), possessing the gene would be more of an indicator of risk, and not a guarantee of future alcoholic offspring. So, while the nature side of the nature vs. nurture debate may be picking up steam, the kind of parent you are is obviously way more important than your genetic legacy, whether you're talking about alcoholic tendencies or hair color.

Without a doubt, and regardless of your family history, when it comes to safeguarding your future children from becoming heavy drinkers, the single best thing you can do is model good behavior for them. That means enjoying alcohol in a controlled way, and encouraging your kids to do the same once they've reached the legal drinking age.

Q: *"This may sound silly, but what about my husband's, uh, contribution? He was drunk as a skunk when we conceived. Could his sperm have been affected?"*

Your husband and his liquor-loving ways are an excellent note to close on. In men, alcohol is well-known for its positive effect on libido and its negative effect on performance, but the jury's still out on precisely how much—and even if—paternal exposure to alcohol affects fertility and the health of babies. (It certainly isn't as clear-cut as it is for women, to say the least.)

The current thought is that light to moderate drinking (up to three drinks a day) in men doesn't appear to do much harm to the sperm, although prolonged and heavy alcohol exposure has been shown to have a negative effect on testosterone, as well as sperm count, quality, and motility. To put your mind at ease, a spermie that's strong enough to find and fertilize an egg is generally in good shape to begin with. So we feel confident saying no—a drunk dad at the time of conception will likely not lead to problems and definitely cannot cause disorders like Fetal Alcohol Syndrome.

But now that you are pregnant—and there's always a but—both you and your partner are best off heading down the sober path to parenthood together. It took the two of you to create that kid, and it'll take the two of you to stray strong for each other during tough times ahead. Now more than ever, the sober, sympathetic shoulders of your significant other can help bear some of the burden you're carrying, both in your belly and between your ears.

chapter

2

THE FIRST-TRIMESTER BLUES:

Withdrawal, Work, and Keeping It Under Wraps

"I'd only had one drink, but I was
sick as a dog the next day. Suddenly, it
occurred to me that it probably wasn't a
hangover—it was morning sickness!"
—*Tara C., 36, Atlanta, GA*

Welcome to the first trimester—you'll feel hungover all the time without ever having drunk a drop. If you're really lucky, you won't even *want* any alcohol at this stage. And when your tummy does trouble you, at least you'll be in good company: up to 70 percent of moms-to-be experience morning sickness at some point during their pregnancies. But since it really rears its ugly head any time of the day—happy hour included!—that normally noisome nausea can make for quite an able accomplice in quelling any rogue Cosmo cravings. However, for a great many of us, the desire to drink supercedes the urge to purge, at least occasionally, during those first few months.

But abstain you must, and unless you had the foresight to embark on a nice, leisurely withdrawal plan during those months you spent trying to conceive, it's not like you've got the time to take it slowly—now that you know you're knocked up, booze is banned. As in, cold turkey—*ice*-cold turkey. So not only must you immediately adapt to all the other little blessings bestowed by the first trimester—the achy boobs, churning stomach, frequent urination, constant constipation, and chronic exhaustion, as well as adjusting to the fact that *you are actually going to be somebody's mother* in roughly six to nine months—getting used to sudden and absolute alcohol abstinence is an unwelcome prospect for most. Though we can't make the pain go away entirely, there are ways to ease your transition from good-time gal to sober sister.

First of all, it is absolutely critical that the Newly Non-Drinking Girl limit the amount of stress she faces during the tricky first trimester. One way to do this is to address the secondary fallout generated by that most delicate of conditions—the combination of early pregnancy and sobriety. In other words, aside from the unpleasant physical and psychological crap you're already dealing with, you'll need to learn how to adequately manage loads of external pressure, too. This comes namely in the form of other people, and the social, familial, and professional strain they heap upon your crowded headspace during this very private, personal time.

The challenge of keeping it quiet is a common source of anxiety in these early days. While some women shout the news from the rooftop the second they pee on that stick (and are therefore able to openly embrace instant sobriety without contending with prying eyes or personal questions), most of us choose to employ a bit of discretion during the first trimester. But how do you avert suspicion when you're fondly known as the office lush or resident mixologist among your peers and colleagues?

It's a delicate situation. Of course, the choice is yours—you might decide to let friends and family know but keep it to yourself at work, for a variety of sensitive reasons. Or maybe your superstition and/or pragmatism will have you hiding the good news from just about everyone. Just keep in mind that silence, though golden, is a heavy burden to bear alone, which is why we highly recommend you do at least tell the father. No matter what life throws your way during the next few months, your partner will be your best ally in helping you negotiate the physical and psychological minefield that is the first trimester.

Our advice? Fake it 'til you make it! The drinks in this chapter are old favorites with a new twist (mainly, that they're lacking one), or simply a few tasty ways to make it look like you can still keep up with the gang. That is, of course, until the big news breaks.

'N Tonic

Here's a refreshing and simple variation on an old classic. One of these before bed is also a good way to prevent those killer middle-of-the-night calf cramps that may be plaguing you during your second and third trimesters. (It's the quinine in the tonic water that does it!)

Ice

1 ½ oz. lime juice

Tonic water

Fill highball glass almost to the top with ice. Pour in lime juice and then pour tonic into the glass until it's full. Stir well, and garnish with a wedge of lime.

Cold Turkey Instead of Wild Turkey

Okay, here we go...

Getting used to the sober life, especially when you've quit cold turkey, is bound to be an adjustment...make that *annoyance*. (We're no saints; we realize that none of this sounds very appealing right now!) But just keep your eye on the prize—a happy, bouncing bundle of baby—and we know you won't have any trouble trying sobriety on for size.

We humbly offer up the following suggestions to help ease you through withdrawal, with our sincerest apologies:

Carry a Teetotaling Talisman

Sometimes, turning to a good luck charm in times of temptation can curb a craving long enough to let you leave it in the dust. If a simple stone or religious charm isn't enough, that positive HPT, a swatch of paint or fabric from the nursery you're planning, an early ultrasound photo, or a pacifier are a few we recommend. Carry it around in your purse or pocket and take a peek when you want to party. Now, that's some powerful baby mojo.

Take It One Day at a Time

Though you may have had to quit drinking overnight,

remember that you haven't been handed a life sentence. Get a pregnancy calendar and cross off the days as you go along. Onlookers in on your big secret will be delighted by your eager anticipation of the new arrival, while only you will know the evil truth—that your Due Date is also your Do Date. As in, Do Drink.

Practice Positive Visualization

When visions of daiquiris dance in your head, think about baby and rub your tummy. Sure, it sounds trite, but if you do it often enough, your brain will begin to associate alcohol cravings with your impending motherhood. When that happens, it's unlikely you'll be very tempted to knock back a pint. If you doubt the effectiveness of the technique, ask your partner if he ever thinks about baseball during those special, intimate times when he should be thinking about you.

Perfect the Art of Substitution

The majority of this book is dedicated to the myriad and marvelous things you can do instead of drink while you're pregnant. Try a bunch out and see what works for you, whether it's engaging in an alternate oral fixation, upping your overall health factor, replacing alcoholic rituals with traditions geared more toward temperance, or simply consciously shifting your perspective from loving liquor to living the clean life. You're bound to find a few ways to not only take the edge off, but also enjoy yourself in the process.

Our favorite substitution?

Sugar—in all its perfectly processed glory.

Sugar Rush

Since many pregnant women opt to abstain from, or at least limit, diet soft drinks because of their sketchy nutritional content, choosing to indulge in full-sugar cola, ginger ale (perfect for battling first-trimester tummy trouble), and, our new favorite, cream soda (delicious!), is one of the many unexpected, guilt-free benefits of gestational sobriety. Even if you prefer the less sweet flavor of diet soda, getting used to soft drinks the way they were meant to be enjoyed isn't really all that hard.

And there's another plus side: technically, once you give up alcohol, you should have weight loss, so it's up to you to make sure that doesn't happen! Sugar sodas and all their glorious empty calories make the perfect stand-in for the many Cosmos you're no longer drinking. Of course, you *could* do the right thing and replace all that booze with something healthy, but a little unwholesome indulgence every day—whether it comes in the form of soda, chocolate, ice cream, giant muffins, *foie gras,* whipped cream, or anything else your pregnant palate desires—may help keep those far more serious alcohol cravings at bay.

To figure out what you're looking at in terms of pounds saved, here's how it breaks down:

1. First, calculate the daily calories you'd normally consume through alcohol. For example: 165 calories for your favorite drink x 1.5 a day comes in at about 245 calories total (the usual happy-hour cocktail, plus that little somethin'-somethin' to account for those extra few on weekends).

2. Then, come up with a number for your entire pregnancy. So, those 245 calories a day add up to 1,715 calories a week, and 61,740 calories over thirty-six weeks (not forty weeks, since most women find out they're pregnant about one month in).

3. Finally, divide 61,740 by 3,500—the average amount of calories it takes to gain a pound—to figure out how much weight you'd technically lose over thirty-six weeks if you weren't pregnant and gave up alcohol. *That comes to 17.6 pounds!*

But since you *are* pregnant, and the point is to gain weight, not lose it, you've got all those extra calories to play around with now. And that's *in addition* to the extra 150 to 300 calories per day most experts recommend pregnant women consume.

Now all you have to do is choose how you wanna spend 'em!

Embrace Your New Identity

Though your Old Milwaukee self may not much like your Newly Non-Drinking self, revel in this time. Motherhood, after all, is going to be a very different phase in your life, and how you deal with these sorts of changes will determine just how difficult the adjustment will be. If you can, try to perceive your pregnancy as a bit of a dry run for all the new but ultimately rewarding challenges that lie ahead.

Keeping the News Quiet When the Booze Gives It Away

Both at work and at play, for those who know you and your martini-loving ways, just saying no can be a dead giveaway that something's up. Before you were even pregnant, you may have noticed how friends and family seem to have a strange need to be the first to find out, stealing your thunder faster than you can say "Perrier with lemon, please."

But there's a time to obfuscate, and there's a time to celebrate. If you're not ready to share the good news just yet, there are plenty of ways to prevent the knowing smiles, the suspicious stares, and the rude outbursts. When your sudden abstinence from alcohol raises a red flag, the super strategies we've listed over the next few pages will help you divert any unwanted attention from your personal reproductive processes.

We suggest you employ a combination of these techniques, rotating your excuses and tactics frequently in order to quash any unwelcome questions before they arise. (How many times a month can you have the flu, right?) Sure, it may all seem very cloak-and-daggerish, even outright deceptive at times, but in the spirit of secrecy, anything goes. Your body is your business, and you reserve the right to keep your pregnancy private until the precise moment you choose to reveal it.

Bloody Shame

This is always an excellent choice for a first-trimester fake-your-way-through-cocktail-hour drink. Best of all, the tomato juice totally counts towards reaching that pesky fruit-and-vegetable quota. (If you really need to stretch it, so does the lemon.)

Ice

4 oz. tomato juice

½ tsp. horseradish

½ tsp. Worcestershire sauce

2 or 3 drops Tabasco sauce

Dash lemon juice

Salt and pepper, to taste

Carrot stick

Celery salt and/or celery stick for garnish

Shake all the ingredients together with ice in a cocktail shaker and pour into an old-fashioned glass, rimmed with celery salt if that's the way you like it. Garnish with a celery stick and carrot.

Eight Excellent Excuses for Staying Sober

So here's how to keep that bump of yours from showing up unannounced, whether you're showing yet or not.

1. Suffer from an Imaginary Illness: Lie like a rug

and no one will suspect a thing. Why aren't you drinking? You can't—you're taking medicine. For what? Nothing scary, serious, or contagious. (Allergies, a migraine, or the decidedly benign sinus infection make the perfect fake diseases.) You may want to go so far as to carry a dummy pill bottle filled with some of those horse-pill prenatal vitamins, and make a big show of taking them in front of everybody. In a similar spirit, blame morning sickness on the flu, food poisoning, or even a hangover if you're feeling feisty and ironic.

2. Bring Your Car Everywhere: You could always offer to be the designated driver, in which case your sobriety will be appreciated and not derided. But even if you're just chauffeuring yourself around, only a fool would dare question why you aren't getting wasted when you have to hit the road in half an hour.

3. Just Fake It: Avoid public and/or conspicuous drink ordering. If you're at a restaurant or a table at a club, excuse yourself just as the waiter comes around, then head to the bar yourself later. Come back with something that looks like a rum and Coke.

4. Employ a Wingman: Order the same drink as your spouse/friend-in-the-know and have them double-fist all night. It's lots of fun for them (they'll be twice as drunk!), and nobody will notice that you haven't taken a single sip. Also, check out Chapter 5, "Getting a Social

Life: Birthdays, Barbecues, and Barflies, Oh My!" on page 133, for more tips on surviving social situations without alcohol.

5. Keep the Right Company: Hang around the already-pregnant girl, recovering alcoholic, or any other known abstainer, since people usually expect to see less alcohol in their general vicinity. Not only will their temperance not draw attention to your own, but it will keep your covetous cravings to a minimum.

6. Adopt a New Virtue or Vice: We recommend gossip. It won't hurt the baby, and a little mild rumor-slinging—especially about deserving bosses, unpitiable celebrities, and well-known jerks—will have people focusing on who you're talking about instead of what you're not drinking. You might also want to fake athleticism, religion, or health-food addiction for a while, or pretend to be in training for a triathlon or something like that. If you've already gained forty pounds, this might not fly, but it's always worth a shot if you can pass it off as muscle. When your big news finally hits, you can explain away anything nasty you may have said or done by playing the my-hormones-are-crazy-and-the-first-trimester-is-so-difficult card. It trumps everything.

7. Work That Wardrobe Magic: If you're the protruding sort who starts showing the second you pee positive, keeping your burgeoning belly under wraps poses a logistical problem when you're trying to keep things on the down-low. Pull a Sarah Jessica Parker on *Sex and the City* and carry strategically placed shopping bags, newspapers, coats, file folders, and any prop you can think of. Play cold and wear an oversized sweater all the time. Keeping it monotone, layered, and loose also helps hide the beginnings of a bump. If all else fails and you notice someone sizing up your stomach, you have two options:

1) Eat enormous amounts of chocolate in public and complain about how you haven't been able to make it to the gym in weeks.

2) Loudly curse your steroidal allergy medication/birth control pills/newly diagnosed thyroid condition for making you so damn bloated.

8. Opt for Full Disclosure Early On: Crazy as it may sound, being up-front about trying to conceive may raise a few eyebrows at first, but people will quickly absorb the information and move on, especially if you warn them you won't be telling them until after the three-month mark anyway when and if you do get knocked up. As you continue to eschew alcohol, folks will continue to assume you're still just trying, so imagine their surprise when you announce that you're actually due in twenty minutes.

Note: This approach is probably most appropriate for close friends instead of colleagues (whose lives might be adversely affected by your pregnancy) or distant family members (Great Aunt Lulu's been on your case to have kids for years, so encouraging her may up the annoyance factor considerably when she suggests maybe you aren't doing it right).

Cranberry Mocktail

It's easy to fake it with this easy-to-drink classic, since it's impossible to tell the nonalcoholic version from the real thing just by looking at it. Just whisper in the bartender's ear to ix-nay the odka-vay and you'll fit right in. Boozeless bonus: you'll also be fending off those nasty urinary tract infections so many of us are prone to during pregnancy. Aren't cranberries cool?

Ice

5 oz. cranberry juice

3 oz. soda water

Fill a highball glass with ice and pour the cranberry juice in. In case you're using a different type of glass or don't have a measuring cup, it's about ⅔ of the way with the cran, or even halfway if you like your drink less "juicy." Add soda water (until it fills the glass) and garnish with a wedge of lime.

The War at Work

Though the inconvenience posed at work by you selfishly deciding to have a family isn't worth losing more than, say, three nights' sleep over, you have every reason and every right in the world to keep it to yourself for now. While we all know the problems and discrimination faced by working moms, many of us feel that there's also a sneaking bias out there against women *without* kids—namely, the fear that we're going to have some and screw up everything for everyone else.

Obviously, that bean you're brewing is going to be somebody's client someday, but only the most enlightened of bosses will have the prescience to appreciate your current condition as a contribution to the future of the business world. Sadly, most of them will simply see your beautiful babe as a thorn in their side. Don't let that suck all the fun out of it for you. Nobody on their deathbed ever wished they'd spent more time at the office, and you have a right to become a mom *and* make the necessary adjustments in your professional life in order to do so.

Still, we are living in the real world, and the longer you can keep things quiet, the easier it might be on everyone, provided you're not the guilty type. Maybe your supervisor and/or coworkers are asses, and you fear nine long months of repercussions, discrimination, and judgment. Or maybe you're worried that *you're* the one being the jerk—as in, perhaps you were only hired last month and feel a bit sheepish about your little lamb coming along so soon. Even when the timing at work's just right, you may be just plain superstitious, or want to wait to tell anyone until after the first trimester when the miscarriage risk goes down. Whatever the case may be, abstaining from alcohol could interfere with your plan to keep it quiet.

Though it may seem odd, when you think about it, drinking often plays a supporting role in the office theater. Liquor is well-known as a business lubricant, and many deals are sealed over a friendly cocktail or two. Similarly, after-hours functions and working lunches and dinners are becoming an ever-increasing part of the job in every field, from accounting to zoology.

And so, some professional adjustment is often necessary for the Newly Non-Drinking Girl. Many of the privacy-protecting strategies we outlined in the previous section, "Keeping the News Quiet When the Booze Gives It Away," are general enough to be useful for work functions, too, and should be zealously employed to keep nosy coworkers in the dark. That said, the office and its various satellite incarnations occasionally present particular conundrums in need of specialized consideration, which we'll discuss on page 63. After your pregnancy is public knowledge, continue to use the following professionally tailored teetotaling techniques, and you're sure to sail through the stormy seas of working sobriety as dry as a bone.

Sexless in the City
(aka Virgin Manhattan)

A sexless night in your city would have kept you from having to turn down real drinks to begin with, right? Oh well. You might as well celebrate your current state with what many say is a dead-ringer for the whiskeyful original. Jury's still out.

Ice

¼ cup cranberry juice

¼ cup orange juice

1 tsp. maraschino cherry juice

¼ tsp. lemon juice

9 dashes orange bitters

Add ingredients to your cocktail shaker and shake, shake, shake. Strain into a chilled cocktail glass, or serve on the rocks in an old-fashioned glass. Garnish with a couple of maraschino cherries, or five or six if you can't help yourself.

Party Planning

As the eggnog starts to flow, people's tongues start to wag. If they notice you're not partaking, you'll be the topic of conversation all night. So now's the time to try out a few of our Eight Excellent Excuses for Staying Sober on page 55. The goal at work functions, as always, is to keep the focus off you and, therefore, off your fertility.

Here are our favorite tactics for deflecting unwanted attention from curious colleagues, as well as a few big no-nos if you don't want to raise suspicions:

1. Always have an ambiguously shaded drink in your hand: Soda—brown or clear, and with a wedge of something citrusy—can stand in for any number of real alcoholic beverages. Make sure it's always nearly full, lest that well-meaning chap from accounting ask to freshen it up for you.

2. Start a rumor or spread a vicious lie the instant someone's eyes dart to your burgeoning bump: "Did you hear they might be merging the Toledo and Akron branches?" or "Is it true the CEO hired that boy from the mailroom to clean his pool this summer?"

3. Bore everybody into leaving you alone: One of the easiest ways to clear a room at a work party is to talk about the job. Ask a few coworkers if they think company forecasts for the third quarter might be a little ambitious, or whether anyone knows if the exception to

Subsection 3.2 under Clause D of the company's HMO policy handbook might be applicable to any nonresident aliens related to you by blood and living in your household.

4. Complain loudly about menstrual cramps: Pop a fake Midol and nobody will think you're pregnant, nor will they expect you to chase it down with a rum and Coke.

5. Unless you're ready to break the news, *never*, under any circumstances, should you complain about or even *discuss* the following topics while socializing with coworkers:

- Nausea
- Lack of onsite corporate day care facility
- Bone-crushing exhaustion, the likes of which you've before never experienced
- The ticking of your biological clock
- The federal government's unwillingness to initiate a paid maternity-leave plan
- Other people's babies, regardless of how cute or how fresh out of the womb (the glint in your eye might give it away)

Now for the easy part. Above all else, alcohol is also the great equalizer. It really loosens everyone up, so once you've secured your alcohol-free perimeter, you're ready to focus on the best thing about being sober at a work party: all that access to the inside track—and being clear-headed enough to take advantage of it for a change. Simply wait until your boss is finished making out with the janitor 'neath the mistletoe, then hit her up for whatever it is you've been dreaming of. Later on, no self-respecting person in a position of power would dare admit she was too drunk to remember approving your request for the empty corner office or to attend that conference in Maui.

Unexpected bonus once you're showing: you can enjoy the party without being hit on by suddenly uninhibited supervisors and coworkers, since the belly acts as a buffer. For once, the Monday-morning-after-the-Friday-before won't be an awkward nightmare.

Business Trips and Traps

Lots of bosses actually hire people based on who they'd like to hang out with at a hotel or airport bar. So what do you do when you're suddenly no longer the good-time gal your coworkers are counting on to liven up a boring out-of-town meeting or long layover? Just chalk it up to personal problems, of course! Make up something harmless, like a mentally ill cousin or an on-the-verge-of-divorce stepsister, and people will understand why you're not in a partying mood. Warn them on the way over that you're going to be a downer, so that any expectations of long, lingering drinks and late nights will be kept to a minimum. A rotating combination of other excuses—illness, exhaustion, covert mocktail substitutions, and so on—will also help crush any questions arising from your newly sober stylings.

Socializing with Clients

There are people out there who sincerely do not trust those who do not drink; similarly, many clients and/or associates expect a certain amount of friendly shmoozing and boozing to take place while business matters are being attended to. No matter what stage in the negotiations you're at, keep their glasses full full full, because the drunker they get, the less likely they'll be to notice what you're doing, *and* the better chance you'll have of bending them to your will. Then, at the proverbial nineteenth hole, after you've finally reeled in that big fish and you can't very well turn down a toast to your new venture together, you've got to fake it like you've never faked it before: knock back three martini glasses full of water and olives, cry big wet tears when you tell them you're allergic to champagne, subtly spill your Sidecar into a potted plant, and if all else fails, fake a phone call from a family member with "bad news." Whatever it takes...

Virgin Lime Rickey

This virgin classic is all about lime—the one dedicated ingredient that's virtually synonymous with "cocktail."

Ice

1 dash grenadine

1 oz. lime juice

6 oz. club soda, or to fill

Pour lime juice into a highball glass filled with ice. Top with club soda and stir. Add grenadine and stir again. Garnish with a wedge of lime.

Liquid Lunches and Drinking Dinners

Deadlines have no regard for your delicate condition. The frustration/exhaustion of having to work though lunch or dinner or into the wee hours is often mediated by a beer or bottle, and now that you're pregnant it's doubly hard to both stay awake *and* suffer through it all without any mood-altering liquids. If it doesn't happen often, you can play sick once or twice and leave it at that—it's not a lie since you probably really *do* feel like crap, anyway. But the last thing you want is to be the one to beg out early all the time, since people's opinions are formed on the spot and they may not extend you the courtesy of retroactive forgiveness once you reveal the real reason for your absence or abstinence in a few months' time. So just order a coffee instead—don't worry, a little bit of caffeine just this once won't be bad for baby, especially considering what the alternative is—and say that you prefer to stay sharp to get the job done, and that you'll celebrate at home later by getting some sleep. Your boss will appreciate your dedication when you show up early tomorrow morning bright-eyed and bushy-tailed.

For a formerly lucky few, working through lunch over a bottle of wine might be the rule rather than the exception. So how do you keep your pregnancy to yourself when you're suddenly turning down drinks on a daily basis? In situations like these, you may simply have to say something like, "I've decided to cut back on the hooch for a while." Keep it vague, but stay firm. Whether they chalk it up to alcoholism, pregnancy, or the South Beach Diet, people may rib you about it at first, or even apply full-on pressure, but eventually they'll get the idea, see that you're serious, and move on, provided they're not still in high school.

Classic Shirley Temple

We know. You could have thought of this one on your own since you've been drinking them since you were, like, three. But they're worth rediscovering for their copious amounts of ginger ale—the key to nausea relief. Ordering one at a social event is a real conversation-starter. You might get some sideways glances, too, though you're guaranteed to score some smirks in the humor department, whether your big news is out yet or not.

Ice

1 oz. grenadine

6 oz. (ish) ginger ale

Orange slices and maraschino cherries, for garnish

Fill a collins or highball glass with ice. Add grenadine and fill the glass to the top with ginger ale. Garnish with a maraschino cherry (or five or six) and an orange slice.

Morning Sickness Makeover

It ain't easy being queasy. Puking in the privacy of your own home is one thing, but if you suddenly get swept away by a wave of nausea at work, hiding it may be more difficult, especially with the legions of nosy coworkers surrounding you at all times. Your best defense here is a good offense, so swing your bowl time into further proof of your hard-partying ways and blame it on a hangover! You could end up with a reputation as the office lush, but that may be preferable to admitting baby's on board this early on in the game. Pack it in and go home early for added impact.

A word of warning: if you've got severe morning sickness and spend more time doubled over the bowl than at your desk, blaming booze too often will likely land you an intervention, when all you really wanted was a baby shower just a few months down the line. So if you know you tend to get sick at a certain time of day, anticipate in advance and visit a bathroom far, far away. For those who work in closer quarters, learn how to puke quietly and carry a big breath mint.

Leaving the Lush Life

Are you the office souse? In some ways, having a reputation as a party girl might help, not hurt, your chances of maintaining the mystery. When people are used to seeing you come in late or nap at your desk, they may just assume you had another crazy night. Little do they know you slept fourteen hours and still can't keep your eyes open without toothpicks. Continue to regale your jealous coworkers with tales of your amazing tolerance for tequila, and then have a good laugh about it when you finally come out of the conception closet.

In closing, however, we sincerely recommend that you stay as focused as possible when it comes to work.

Because when the truth is at last revealed, the sad fact is that most people will expect your mind to turn to mush just because you're pregnant. Don't give them the satisfaction—stay strong and work as hard as you can for as long as you can. Hopefully, it'll earn you some consideration later on when you're too big to move or think, and have a doctor's appointment every two days.

Absolutely Not
(aka End Wrench)

Absolutely not a screwdriver, that is. We were shocked to discover how remarkably this one tastes like the real thing— that tonic bite at the end is sort of similar to the way the original version's vodka tingles on the tongue. You can vary the amount of tonic to suit your taste, and it also helps to let the drink sit for a few minutes to let the tonic mellow.

Ice

1 ½ oz. tonic water

6 oz. (ish) orange juice

Cherries, for garnish

First, fill a highball glass with ice. Pour in the tonic and then fill the glass to the top with orange juice. Stir with a swizzle stick and garnish with a cherry.

Surviving the Perfect Storm of Sobriety: When a Positive HPT, a Business Trip, and Morning Sickness Collide

I can see that second line on the FRED (First Response Early Detection test, for you newbies out there) faintly appearing before my very eyes. I choke down the rest of my Diet Coke, instantly realizing it will probably be my last for a while. *Is it true?* I ask myself. *Am I really pregnant?* Second time around doesn't mean the denial's any less profound, I guess. The real kicker is, with a toddler running around, giving up alcohol for the next nine months is going to be even harder.

The timing couldn't be crazier. If ever there were a Perfect Storm of pregnancy-induced sobriety, I'd be heading straight into it. Serves me right, I suppose, for peeing on a stick in an airport bathroom. You see, I'm about to board a plane for Stockholm to enjoy what I *thought* would be the biggest boozefest of the year. The four-day work conference with colleagues would be loaded with alcohol-related recreation, and now, not only won't I be drinking, but I'm actually the organizer of the final event—a huge party at one of the Seven Wonders of the Drinking World, Absolut's very own Icebar. The walls, the barstools, the glasses, even the *art* in this legendary establishment are carved entirely out of crystal-clear ice shipped in from northern Sweden's Torne River.

Sh*t. Now what?

Okay, here's how it goes down...

I arrive safely in Stockholm. Surprisingly, I feel okay, even though I hardly slept on the plane. (I nearly had a stroke when I realized that with baby now on board, my trusty Ambien was suddenly off-limits for the seven-hour overnight flight, to say nothing of my usual vodka chaser...) Mother guilt creeps in again at the airport after I order an extra-strong black coffee and just stare at it, bleary-eyed, for a while. *I need to drink it...I am going to drink it...* and I do.

Ah, that all-too-familiar first-trimester fear. When that kicks in, the denial phase is over and you basically hold your breath till the milestone of week thirteen, when, of course, there's a whole new world of worries to contend with. For now, though, I need to figure out exactly how I'll survive the next four days.

By the time I check in to the hotel, exhaustion hits hard. Is it the time difference? The lack of sleep? My first pregnancy symptom? No matter—I can't let it slow me down. There's too much to do. So, what next? Should I tell somebody or keep it totally to myself? I pretty much always warned everyone that if my wine glass was empty, then most likely my uterus was full. So, will they notice? Should I fake it? I'd really prefer not to let my colleagues in on my little secret until the timing is right for all of us. My head is spinning...

But with the storm of extenuating circumstances brewing overhead and no lifeboat in sight, I realize there's no way I can survive it alone. So I make a calculated decision to recruit Stephanie—a friend, colleague, and perfect ally, since, as luck would have it, she's pregnant and out of the closet about it. Misery loves company, I remind myself, and share my wonderful (if untimely!) news with her as my stomach churns for what certainly won't be the last time. Instead of being shocked, she gives me a knowing smile, and I realize I must look as crappy as I feel. More important, though, Stephanie offers her unconditional support and discretion. For the first time since I peed on that stick, I feel safe and calm.

As the days swing from conference sessions to restaurants and bars and back again, I'm further relieved to realize that the hiding part isn't nearly as bad as I'd imagined. I suspect nobody suspects, and it turns out, for whatever reason, that people don't seem to be imbibing as much as I thought they'd be. Maybe they're lightweights, or, more likely, I never really bothered noticing their drinking habits before. And because of that, it occurs to me that they probably aren't monitoring mine, either. And so, my orders of sparkling water, juices, and sodas raise no alarm bells, of either pregnancy, former alcoholism, or temperance. Even the culmination of the trip—the closing party at Icebar—goes off without a hitch, and I'm too busy having fun and staying on top of everything to mourn the loss of my usual martinis.

Back home, I draw on my positive experience in Stockholm for the rest of my first trimester. If I survived that, I tell myself, I can easily go without drinking in the controlled environment of more familiar surroundings for as long as it takes. Unlike when I was pregnant with my first kid, I decide the route to go this time is full-on disclosure to friends. Lucky for me, with an eighteen-month-old already at home, it's not like I'm going out much anyway these days.

Though I'm proud to have weathered the Perfect Storm without a single drop of alcohol, I must admit that I sometimes feel like I missed out a little. I mean, how often does one have the opportunity to visit as venerable a drinking establishment as the one I gave the cold shoulder to in Stockholm? So, whenever I think about all those excellent, icy drinks not drunk, I just remind myself that the bar will be open again when my forty weeks are up.

I wonder…do you think they might have milk martinis for baby on the menu at Icebar?

—C.A.

3

HOMEMADE HAPPY HOUR:

Turn On, Tune In, and Drop Out...Without a Drop

"My husband asked me to fix him a martini after work. I threw a jar of olives at his head instead. How can I stay calm AND sober without killing him...or having a nervous breakdown in the process?"

—*Mandy K., 35, Phoenix, AZ*

We feel your pain. You finally get home after The Day from Hell. You kick off your heels, grab the ice tray, reach for the shaker, and then it hits you like a ton of dirty diapers—you're gestating! That maraschino at the bottom of your usual Manhattan suddenly seems as far away as Mumbai. What to do, what to do?

First of all, stay calm. If you lose your cool, you might also lose your resolve, and we certainly can't have that. But simply putting happy hour in your home on hold for the following forty weeks obviously isn't going to work, either. You *need* to wind down after work, reward yourself with something special. How else can you be expected to banish the office/store/site/classroom to the back of your brain where it belongs for the next twelve to fourteen hours?

Contrary to what you may believe, there *are* ways to wind down without a drink. Actually, we've come up with ten—each one designed to bring physical and mental peace to your place. (We'll discuss how to handle situations out in the field in Chapter 5: "Getting a Social Life: Birthdays, Barbecues, and Barflies, Oh My!")

We firmly believe that if you have a list of gratifying nonalcoholic happy-hour alternatives to draw on, and your home is well-stocked with the necessary equipment and accouterments, you (and your husband's skull) should make it through your pregnancy just fine. So make like a Girl Guide from now on and Be Prepared.

In this chapter, our offerings run from the juicy to the hot, with a little fizzy and sweet in between. Get creative, have fun, and make 'em any way you like 'em—it's your happy hour!

Post–Sex on the Beach

Ah, Sex on the Beach. It may be your favorite pre-pregnancy drink, or it may just be what got you into this mess in the first place. Either way, raise your glass and toast to the good old days…

Ice

1 part orange juice

1 part cranberry juice

1 oz. peach nectar

1 tsp. grenadine

Cherries, for garnish

Fill a highball glass almost to the rim with ice. Pour in one part orange juice and one part cranberry juice (roughly 3 oz. of each). Pour in 1 oz. peach nectar. Stir well and add grenadine on top. Garnish with a cherry (heh, heh). This may also be shaken in a cocktail shaker and strained into a martini or shooter glass.

Variation: Substitute the peach nectar with pear nectar for a "Regrets on the Beach."

Ten New Happy-Hour Habits

Nine months is a long, long time, and it's important to feel like you're not depriving yourself. The key, as we said, is to replace your pre-pregnancy after-work habits with a relaxing new ritual or two. Anything goes, so long as it fulfills the basic premise of happy hour—shifting gears through self-indulgence and/or mood-altering activities. Remember, it's not about working out or keeping your hands busy; distraction from any alcoholic fantasies you may be having is simply not enough. What you need now is pure, unadulterated, pain-free recreation to look forward to on a nightly basis.

1. Like a Virgin!

By far, the easiest way to replace your beloved old drink is with a beloved new drink. The alcohol-free mocktail recipes scattered throughout the pages of this book are a good place to start, or feel free to experiment with various formulations of your own.

Note: Any drink worth its celery salt deserves a proper presentation, whether it's a simple highball glass for a lowly Shirley Temple or a half-pineapple hull for a Virgin Bahama Mama. As long as your concoction of choice promotes the concept of Drink as Event, it should work rather well. So boring diet sodas and screwdrivers minus the vodka are out; elaborate preparations involving entire coconuts or dry ice are in.

Shopping list: Appropriate barware, blenders, shakers, and so on, depending on what your poison is. Invest in the proper ingredients too, like nonalcoholic mixers and a selection of those high-quality flavored Italian syrups. The importance of details like cherries, citrus wedges, mini-umbrellas, and sugared rims cannot be overstated.

Protruding Navel

Here's our nod to one of the best girlie drinks ever—the Fuzzy Navel. We renamed it in honor of one of the grossest physical aspects of pregnancy, though if you tend to lean toward the hirsute while you're expecting, feel free to call it a Fuzzy Tummy. Whatever works for you.

Ice

2 oz. peach nectar

6 oz. orange juice

Orange slices, for garnish

Fill highball glass almost to the top with ice. Pour the peach nectar first, and then the orange juice into the glass, stir well, and garnish with an orange slice.

2. Soak It Out

Draw a bath often enough and pretty soon, it'll be the one drawing you! The many blessings bestowed by a good, long soak have been employed by various civilizations for millennia in the fight against stress, dirt, and disease. Indeed, the heady combination of soap or salts and warm water rivals even booze for its miraculous ability to melt away the day, to say nothing of the temporary weightlessness it affords your gravid frame.

If your partner happens to get home before you do every day, leave standing instructions for him to have things ready for when you walk in the door. (If your schedule is erratic, give him a ten-minute warning call.) If you have to run your own bath, set things up in the morning so all you need to do after work is hit the tap and hop in. Just make sure the water temperature is warm, not hot—especially during your first trimester—and get ready to get pruney.

Shopping list: Scented candles, possibly some ambient music, a good neck pillow, a super-luxe bathrobe, and the best products you can afford in terms of oils, salts, bubbles, and after-bath lotions and creams.

3. Feed Your Foot Fetish

When you want to whet your whistle, try wetting your feet instead. It doesn't take full-body submersion to enjoy the relaxing benefits of a bath—a good below-the-knees soak will wash your worries away, whether you work on your feet or not. In fact, those who ride a desk all day will quickly grow to love the process, since swelling during pregnancy makes those fabulous office-chic stacked heels even more of a pain. But the best is yet to come: after twenty minutes or so, towel off those toesies, hand your partner the peppermint foot lotion, and put his hands to work massaging your metatarsals.

Shopping list: A big bowl, some soaking salts or soap, hot tap water, and the very best foot cream you can find.

Nursery Fizz

This simple, fantastic Fizz is a winner in the battle against morning sickness. Though traditionally this drink is made with soda and gin, or even sloe gin, ginger ale stands in here as a worthy and sweet substitute. It also makes for a very handy variation on a mimosa.

Ice

3 oz. ginger ale

3 oz. orange juice

1 splash simple syrup, or a pinch of powdered sugar

Cherries and orange slices, for garnish

Fill a large wine glass with ice and pour in all the ingredients. Garnish with a cherry and an orange slice.

Variation: If the OJ is too tough on your tummy, substitute lemonade instead.

4. Honor Thine Hors d'Oeuvres

Sure, it definitely indulges those oral fixations that have been dogging you, but what's wrong with that? Hors d'oeuvres are an excellent way to use up the 150 to 300 extra calories a day your pregnant body so needs and deserves. Whether the intoxicating scent of baking phyllo pastry brings you back to your brother's Bar Mitzvah in '89, or reminds you more of gallery openings and vernissages, there's always something elegant about finger foods and tiny stuffed thingies.

Remember to keep things fancy, but fun: hors d'oeuvres are more than a snack, they're an event—a formal end to your cubicle-cramped day, served up on a silver tray. That means no crackers out of the box or a cupful of old carrot sticks, 'kay?

Shopping list: You can do it yourself with frozen canapés from your local grocer, order some from a real caterer and freeze them so they're ready to go at a moment's notice, or perhaps whip some up yourself if you're feeling creative and enjoy spending time in the kitchen.

5. Read for Reward

Very few vices are fair game for the mama-to-be. While most would consider reading a virtue, the written word *can* be quite intoxicating, provided you have the right material on hand. Celebrity and/or fashion worship, for example, is among life's little venial sins—naughty, trivial, and readily accessible in about a million magazine pages per week. Similarly, curling up after work with a good romance or chick-lit novel rivals only sleep and alcohol for sheer escapism.

Best of all, reading is decidedly nonteratogenic. In other words, taking the *Shopaholic* series for a spin or researching Sienna Miller's latest choices in handbags will in no way harm your growing baby (though it may hurt your wallet). If you must, an actual novel with some literary merit may be substituted, but choose wisely: that tragic tome endorsed by Oprah's Book Club may leave you more melancholic than lighthearted.

Shopping list: Subscriptions to: *Us Weekly* (the best for celeb baby-bump watching), *People* (for a smattering of feel-good stories), *InStyle* (for what to wear once you get your body back), *In Touch* (heavy on all things plastic-surgical), *Jane* (for sassy, unsilly stories and style), *Cosmopolitan* and *Glamour* (excellent lip gloss reviews and sex tips), and *Vogue* (the utmost in excess as spectator sport). Actual tabloids like *Star* and the *National Enquirer* are loads of gossipy fun, but they'll leave your fingertips filthy and your conscience filthier. As for books, the racier the better—try anything set in antebellum Natchez or Mississippi, or something with a cartoonish Cosmopolitan on the cover.

Afterglow

Who needs rum? A tropical trio of fruit juices lends this mocktail a taste of the exotic, perhaps reminiscent of that honeymoon cruise you took to the Caribbean. This one's equally good blended with a little crushed ice. So kick off those heels, collapse onto the couch, and close your weary eyes…can't you hear those steel drums already?

Ice (cubes or crushed)

1 part grenadine

1 part orange juice

1 part pineapple juice

Cherries and orange slices, for garnish

Fill a highball glass almost to the top with ice. Pour grenadine, orange juice, and pineapple juice into the glass, stir well, and garnish with a skewered orange slice and cherry.

6. Slip into Some Silk

Nobody can relax when they feel like a trussed turkey. In your pre-pregnancy life, putting on your PJs at 6 p.m. might have seemed ridiculous. Not anymore. The instant you rip off those work clothes, you'll instantly settle into a different state of mind. No matter how comfortable the sales girl at the maternity store swore that suit would be, the pea in your pod just needs to be free. Plus, once unencumbered by your professional attire, you may even be inspired to get to bed at a decent hour and catch up on your sleep (which, truth be told, is your one remaining chance for actually escaping reality).

So, as your waistline expands and that waistband tightens, you'll do well to appreciate the fact that nothing—not even a forbidden Fuzzy Navel—will feel as good as slipping into something a little more drawstringed.

Can we get an amen?

Shopping list: Now is not the time to be close to your money. Give it up for cashmere in the winter, silk in the summer. And invest in some appropriate unmentionables, too: ditch the underwire after work for an unflattering but far comfier sports bra or, if your nipples can bear it, no brassiere at all.

7. Get Cooking

A busy career woman like you is probably used to takeout or frozen fare during the week, but cooking a meal from scratch can be quite relaxing. The Zen-like trance induced by chopping vegetables and the sense of accomplishment you'll derive from a supper well served may be enough to take your mind off mixed drinks. If you're used to cooking with a glass of wine by your side, simply substitute a marvelous mocktail of your choosing.

The only caveat we'll include is that if you cook, You-Know-Who must agree to clean up. Otherwise, it's work, and we certainly can't endorse any happy-hour hobby that involves hard labor. There will be plenty of that for you soon enough, along with fewer opportunities to enjoy a candlelit meal and some adult conversation.

Shopping list: Make your grocery list at work and pick up fresh ingredients on the way home, or do the shopping on Sunday for the whole week if that suits you better. Also, we recommend putting whatever you make on a pretty plate—a beautifully set table makes even those less-than-stellar efforts more appealing.

Snips and Snails and Puppy-Dog Tails
(That's what little boys are made of!)

Hair of the dog is often just the thing for a hangover. Though your headaches these days aren't alcohol-induced, they are definitely just as annoying. In that spirit, this mocktail is designed to manage your maternity migraines, thanks to a helpful kick of sugar and caffeine. Also enjoy it post-delivery for an energy boost while dealing with even the rowdiest little guy.

Ice

1 oz. chocolate syrup

1 oz. coffee syrup

1 oz. milk, or splash of half-and-half

3 oz. cola

Cherries, for garnish

First, chill a highball glass by putting it in the refrigerator. Then mix all the ingredients together in a cocktail shaker, pouring the milk in last. Serve over plenty of ice in your chilled glass with a cherry for garnish.

Variation: If you're into it, use diet cola instead—when it comes to virgin drinks, some temperance aficionados claim that artificial sweetener mimics the taste of alcohol better than real sugar does.

8. Write It Down

Even if you've never written anything but a check before, keeping a journal is something everyone should try at least once. It's actually quite easy, and it works like this: you take all your worries and stresses and hopes and dreams for you and your unborn baby, and you put them down on the page. It's cathartic, it's creative, and it's going to free up some much-needed space between your ears. (No need to be self-conscious; nobody's ever going to read it.) So slip in your favorite CD, flop down on the couch, and put pen to paper…

Shopping list: Get thee to a good stationery store and splurge on a beautifully bound journal. Save the Bic for the grocery list and break out that dusty Mont Blanc you got for graduation, because a pretty pen always helps keep the words flowing smoothly.

9. Be a TiVo Diva

What's your guilty pleasure—*Oprah? Days of Our Lives? The View? A Baby Story?* Don't be embarrassed and don't make excuses—sometimes it's okay to like really bad things. Making a regular date with yourself to catch up on all 312 *Survivor* episodes is good, clean fun and an excellent way to shift gears. We don't care who's on the phone or how much your significant other needs you. You and your bowl of popcorn are not to be disturbed.

Shopping list: An electronic recording device of some kind. If TiVo's a no-go, download it and burn it, baby. Or, if you're still clawing your way into the twenty-first century, one of those antique VCRs will actually work quite well for this sort of thing.

Sugar and Spice and Everything Nice (That's what little girls are made of!)

Sure, it'd be nice with real brandy, but this sweet hot toddy still makes a cordial complement to a cold winter's night. It's also a pretty good way to clear out those stuffy sinuses or even relieve a case of insomnia.

1½ cups apple cider or apple juice

½ teaspoon cinnamon

½ teaspoon imitation brandy extract (available in baking section of grocery stores)

1 teaspoon cloves

1 teaspoon grated orange peel

2 teaspoons brown sugar

In a small pot over medium–low heat, combine all ingredients and simmer for twenty minutes. Strain, and serve immediately in a large mug with a cinnamon swizzle stick, if you've got one.

10. Don't Hesitate to Meditate

The quest for inner quiet by focusing the mind may very well be the Newly Non-Drinking Girl's Nirvana. Yes, a self-imposed time-out is arguably *better* than booze when it comes to mastery over your stress. Just open yourself to what billions of people across the globe have known for centuries, and you too could be on the path to peace. Do a little online research or visit a bookstore to find a type of meditation that appeals to you.

Transcendental Meditation, or TM, is the meat-substitute and potatoes of the New Age set, and was marketed during the 1960s as a way to achieve "serenity without drugs." Other religious takes on meditation include Buddhist, Hindu, Jain, Islamic, Taoist, and even some monastic Christian methods. Biofeedback—the electronic monitoring of bodily processes and one's subsequent attempt to exert control over them—can be considered a form as well, as can various psychological relaxation techniques and self-hypnosis.

Of course, formal methods are just fine, but you may find all you really need to induce a Zen-like state is to go up onto the roof for half an hour each day after work and stare out at the city. If you prefer, wander half a mile into the woods, if you've got 'em, and find a quiet clearing you can call your very own for the next thirty minutes. Hell, even a splintering park bench will do the trick. Now make like the Buddha and don't move a muscle...

Shopping list: A mat, some candles, maybe some incense, and a good inflatable doughnut to sit on, if going lotus-style doesn't suit your blossoming hemorrhoids. Several secular meditation methods may call for specific equipment, like biofeedback machines or CD players. Alternately, altars and their attendant gongs, beads, lingams, and multi-armed statuary are nice, but never necessary. However you choose to get quiet, make sure to designate a special space for yourself, free of distracting clutter and other reminders of your worldly life.

Innocent Passion

We know its title is somewhat of an oxymoron, which is why we threw in the pomegranate juice instead of the cranberry that appears in the original recipe. Sometimes, you need a third party to help mix things up—and with baby along for the ride, that shouldn't be too hard to understand these days.

Ice

4 oz. mango-passionfruit juice or syrup, if you can find it

1 dash pomegranate juice

1 dash lemon juice

Club soda

Cherries, for garnish

Fill a highball glass with ice and mix fruit juice, pomegranate juice, and lemon juice. Top off with club soda. Stir well and garnish with a cherry and a long straw.

But What If?

Pregnancy is a beautiful time…some of the time. Yes, you love your little bean already—and hopefully also the person who planted it there—but the pressure, the hormones, and the pain often all add up to something somewhat less than twenty-four-hour joy. And that means things might occasionally get ugly *chez vous*. Home has always been your soft place to land, and when the traditional happy hour treats are suddenly off the menu, old habits die hard, slow, painful deaths.

Here, we address your concerns when it comes to problems abstaining at home.

Q: *"I'm jealous, angry, and tempted because my significant other continues to indulge in happy hour without me."*

These feelings are perfectly normal and by no means make you a bad person, sweetie. They make *him* a bad person. Tell him how you feel, and warn him that you reserve the right to, on occasion, pour his drink down the drain if he dares not abstain right alongside you as a show of support for what you're going through for the sake of your unborn child. Better invest in another inflatable bath pillow, because at your house, abstinence is going to be a group project from now on.

Q: *"I'm all alone, and I fear that without someone else's loving support, or at least their watchful eye, I'll be tempted to knock one back in the privacy of my own home."*

If you're entering into motherhood on your own, either temporarily or permanently, you will need to search your soul for the motivation you need to get through. Get rid of every drop of alcohol in your house, and remember that you're actually *not* alone anymore— you've got baby with you twenty-four hours a day.

Baby Cocktail

Sweet and delicious, just like that bundle of joy that will be joining you shortly. What this lacks in imagination, it makes up for with great taste and convenience. Don't you wish all things baby were this easy?

Ice

2 oz. pineapple juice

2 oz. cream

Pineapple slice, for garnish

Shake ingredients together with ice in a cocktail shaker and strain into a martini glass. Garnish with a pineapple slice.

Q: *"My apartment is a drinker's paradise, from the barstools and Budweiser sign to the amply stocked fridge and pantry. It's driving me nuts!"*

Time to close up shop. Get rid of all the booze, bottles, and related paraphernalia at your place. Out of sight is out of mind, especially when you're on the verge of going out of your head. Whomever you happen to be living with will understand. If not, stab him in the eye with a swizzle stick so he won't be able to see what you're tossing into that trash bag.

Q: *"I tried everything you suggest and my old quitting-time cocktail still beckons seductively, even more so when I'm having a bad day. I'm really worried I'll crack under the pressure."*

Boy, you're a tough case. The ugly truth is, some of us need a little additional help and motivation to get through the times, places, and/or events we most strongly associate with alcohol. Take heart—you're not alone. If you feel this way on a regular basis, or even if you're just having a bad day, Chapters 6 and 7 may be for you. Resources include our very own Twelve-Step Program and plenty of extra inspiration and motivation, as well as the whos and hows of professional sobriety support. The most important thing is that you recognize your feelings, acknowledge their seriousness, and are taking the necessary steps to get that monkey off your back.

4

GETTING HIGH:

Our Four Favorite Fetus-Friendly Ways to Catch a Buzz

"It's amazing how good two Tylenol can feel when you've been substance-free for months!"

—*Kathy D., 30, San Francisco, CA*

You're a healthy, red-blooded woman, swimming in a sea of hormones, and sometimes you simply need to feel the rush of pleasure that comes from, well, some of the more hedonistic aspects of being alive. Alcohol is such an easy way to alter your state of consciousness, but now that the hooch is off-limits, you're going to have to get a little more creative when looking for a safe yet smashing way to escape reality. Even if it's just for a little while, spoiling yourself with the body- and mind-altering methods we outline here will go a long way toward making your alcohol-free pregnancy as pleasantly sinful and self-indulgent as it can be.

As we've stated before, your best chance for success at all this temporary teetotalism is to find alternative forms of stress relief. To that end, we've come up with Our Four Favorite Fetus-Friendly Ways to Catch a Buzz. Each one involves using your own body's hormones and hot spots to attain nirvana, at least for a little while.

All must be entered into cautiously. Since our Fab Four actually boast some fairly impressive physical side effects, we've also included corresponding warnings to draw attention to any situations which, for whatever reason, might lead you to take a pass. Pay extra-close attention—your health and your baby's well-being are at stake.

Sorry, dear. Doctor's orders.

Indulgent, sticky, sensual, caloric...it's going to take something special to replace your old pal alcohol, and the recipes in this chapter have it. Thank heaven this isn't the time to be counting calories.

Sneaky Little Peanut

This addictive little mummy yumminess is not recommended until the start of the nine-month slump (otherwise, you're bound to put on an additional sixty pounds). Even if you can barely move, it's well worth getting up off the couch and breaking out the blender once again. Even better, have that nimble partner of yours do it for you. You're running out of weeks to play the "Help me—I'm pregnant!" card.

1 tbsp. peanut butter

1 oz. chocolate syrup

3 oz. milk

2 scoops vanilla ice cream

Whipped cream, for garnish

Combine first four ingredients in blender and blend until smooth. As always, vary ingredients to your taste. Don't forget the whipped cream—why deprive yourself?

1. Exercise: What an Endorphin or Two Can Do for You

We know you know that exercise is a good thing in general. Well, all the same things apply when you're in a family way. And though it may be more tempting these days to strike up an intimate relationship with your couch instead of your cross-trainers, both your body and your brain will benefit from a few good deeds. Even if you have no idea what an elliptical trainer is, now can be a great time to learn, provided you take things nice and easy and get your doctor's permission first. For you old pros, continuing your regular workout routine—or altering it to suit your new form—is highly recommended.

There's really no end to the saintly virtues of a breaking a good sweat, but during pregnancy, one benefit stands out above all the rest: **endorphins**.

During strenuous exercise, these happy little hormones are released from the pituitary gland into your blood and brain, where they bind with opiate receptors to produce a fantastic buzz. If you're lucky, you're familiar with it already—that great feeling you get during and after an intense workout. Also known as "runner's high," it's a sensation many athletes claim far surpasses alcohol or drugs in terms of its sheer ability to make you blissfully happy.

Wait…did somebody say opiates? Yes, it's true: the release of endorphins has a similar effect to those old opioid standbys, morphine and heroin and opium. Like them, endorphins have a powerful mood-enhancing and pain-killing effect within the brain. But unlike hard drugs, these hormones offer an all-natural buzz; all you have to do to get high is enjoy a good, strong workout. No need to stick a needle in your arm! No need to break out that crazy hookah pipe! Just run and fly!

Three Ways to Work Out

For some, endorphins are an elusive lover. Varying your exercise routine and making sure that it includes the following three components may be the key to enjoying the maximum benefits exercise has to offer.

Cardiovascular training (running, walking, aerobics, swimming, biking—anything that gets your heart rate up) will keep your ticker happy and healthy as it works extra hard over the next forty weeks to circulate your ever-increasing blood volume. (You'll have up to 50 percent more by the time you deliver!) Some of the best forms of cardiovascular exercise during pregnancy include low-impact sports like walking and particularly swimming and water aerobics, which offer the added benefit of temporary weightlessness once your belly blossoms.

Strength training (with weights, bands, machines, or using your own body mass as resistance, from Pilates to push-ups) strengthens bones, joints, and ligaments, and builds muscle—all of which will come in quite handy when that adorable little newborn you're toting around turns from a seven-pound featherweight into a whopping twenty-pounder seemingly overnight. It's also a crucial weapon in the fight against osteoporosis.

Flexibility training (yoga, some Pilates, or simply stretching before and after your workouts) will serve you well during delivery when your knees are up by your shoulders for thirty-six hours straight. Just kidding! (Sort of.) No matter what happens, getting limber will increase blood flow to your muscles and keep your joints and ligaments strong and pliable for the big day and beyond.

Other Inspirational Incentives

Although the aforementioned workout buzz is, we feel, far and away the best reason to get your butt to the gym, it's not the only one. Exercise is a powerful ally in keeping all alcohol at arm's length, as well as many of the other notorious hardships of pregnancy. Best of all, it doesn't take much: most experts agree that the positive benefits of exercise can be achieved in as little as twenty to thirty minutes, three times a week.

Here are a few more plus sides to breaking a sweat during pregnancy.

Control your weight!

You're going to be awfully hungry over the next forty weeks, and now's not the time to deprive yourself in the name of vanity. Sticking to your workout routine is a small price to pay for regular indulgence in chocolate, but more on that later.

Prevent those common pregnancy pains!

Exercise, particularly the aerobic kind, improves circulation—and therefore reduces hemorrhoids, varicose veins, swelling, and muscle cramps—and ups your energy level in general.

Get into great shape for the delivery!

We don't mean to kill your buzz, but they don't call it labor for nothing. The hours you'll spend getting that baby from inside to outside your body will leave you feeling like you've been hit by a truck. The only question that remains is, will it be a pickup or an eighteen-wheeler? Regular exercise might hold the answer, since research suggests that women who work out seem to have shorter labors on average and fewer medical interventions.

Bounce back quicker!

The leaner and meaner your body is now the sooner you'll be up and at 'em after you squirt out that pup.

Not only will you feel better faster if you're in decent shape, but you'll look like a million bucks the whole time. And afterward, those pre-preggers jeans will be sliding up over your hips in no time.

Keep stress and anxiety at bay!
Regular exercise likely reduces your adrenal gland's production of cortisol. Don't worry—that's a good thing, since this steroid has been implicated in the causation of stress. When you work out, you also relieve muscle tension and sleep better. Could you ask for anything more?

It'll make you happy forever!
And we're not just talking about a short-term runner's high. Exercise also increases your levels of serotonin, that bliss-bearing neurotransmitter that all well-balanced brains need in good supply in order to sleep, eat, and be merry. In fact, several significant studies suggest that regular exercise can be as effective as antidepressants in combating depression in the medium and long term. While some antidepressants are considered safe during pregnancy—especially when compared with the risks of serious depression—the fewer drugs you take the better, right? Sweating it out is also a super way to keep postpartum depression at bay, the natural way.

Off-White Russian

This is shockingly delicious and almost tastes like the real thing. It's best enjoyed as an after-dinner drink — especially if you're the designated driver (again!) 'cause there's nothing like the quick kick of caffeine to perk you up for the long trek home.

Ice

1 ½ oz. coffee syrup*

4 oz. whole milk

Fill a rocks glass with ice. First pour in the coffee syrup, then the milk. You could also go with cream for a thicker taste, or choose skim milk for a lighter one, but we like ours with whole. Who's counting calories now, anyway?

Variation: A scoop of vanilla ice cream may be added to pump up this drink's dessert factor.

*To make coffee syrup, use equal parts simple syrup and brewed coffee. Both need to be cold when mixing.

Belly Busters

Before starting or continuing any exercise routine while pregnant, make sure your doctor or midwife knows exactly what you're up to, just in case you're a candidate for restriction; both pre-existing medical conditions and various gestational woes may seriously affect your ability to work out safely.

Aside from that, the following activities are generally not advised during pregnancy:

- **Abdominal workouts:** a little dicey after about twenty weeks, since the baby's weight could prevent adequate blood flow
- **Scuba-diving:** too much pressure, all around
- Contact sports like **football** and **hockey:** save it for after the birth, tough guy
- Anything that involves **lying on your back** or **motionless standing** after the first trimester: again, maintaining adequate circulation is key
- **Weight-lifting:** leave the heavy stuff to those without cervical concerns
- Any activity that takes place six thousand feet above sea level or higher, such as **rock climbing** and **hang gliding**: do we really need to explain this one?
- **Gymnastics, horseback riding, ice skating, downhill skiing,** and **anything else that involves a high likelihood of falling:** protect that burgeoning belly at all costs
- **Ultramarathoning, ironman triathlons,** or **the Tour de France:** while a hardy few may argue otherwise, take a break from the endurance sports
- **Some yoga:** a few of the twistier, more challenging yoga poses might be difficult as your baby bump grows, and ditch **Bikram yoga**—in which you

assume postures in rooms heated to a balmy 105 degrees Fahrenheit—since raising your body temperature is ill-advised during pregnancy

In general, *exercise* good judgment and you should be fine. If you're working out regularly, you also may need to eat a little more than the 150 to 300 extra calories a day recommended for pregnant women. Avoid activities that make you uncomfortable, stay extremely well-hydrated, stick to lower-impact activities as you progress, and if you feel faint, dizzy, or like you may be pushing yourself too hard, stop immediately. The same goes if you're dealing with vaginal spotting or leakage, chest pain, headaches, or anything that doesn't feel quite right. This is the time to stay fit and healthy, not the time to be setting any land-speed records.

2. Spa Treatments: Expensive, Sure, but Absolutely Essential

There is an urban legend circulating out there about a special massage table for pregnant women. This mythical board is padded and soft and scented of lavender, and has two generously sized breast recesses and a giant hole about halfway down through which the preponderance of one's enormous belly can hang free at last. Imagine…sixty to ninety minutes of complete and total relaxation beneath an expert's able hands, combined with a way to lounge oh-so-comfortably on your stomach? Why, it's almost like you're not even pregnant at all! Truth be told, we'd take a good Shiatsu pounding over a mediocre Mai Tai most days of the week; there's simply no better escape. As for the massage table, it's the Hole-y Grail of pregnant pleasure-seekers. But look and ye shall find…

Spa treatments are like the flip side of exercise—all gain and no pain (certain esthetic techniques and deep-tissue massages notwithstanding). You'll look good and feel better after a visit to your friendly neighborhood body shop, since many popular services offer positive physiological benefits, too. And like a good workout, they not only guarantee a fabulous mood in the short term, but will make you feel generally well-kept and looking lovely, especially on those days when you don't feel so hot on the inside.

Mock Champagne #1

Dom it ain't, but that doesn't mean you can't pretend. Like, pretend your breasts don't hurt. Like, pretend your back isn't aching. Like, pretend you can see your feet…You get where we're going with this. Here's the simplest recipe around for this celebratory concoction, since you have enough on your plate already.

2 oz. chilled white grape juice

2 oz. chilled ginger ale

Mix ingredients together in a champagne flute. Pretend.

These Are a Few of Our Favorite Things

Choosing among the facials, mudwraps, manis, pedis, and many glorious massages…ay, *there's* the rub. Though some of the more outlandish health and beauty benefits touted by your local purveyor of bliss can seem like wishful thinking, there's certainly no harm in trying something new. So what if that kukui nut-oil facial isn't really better than Botox, and that Ayurvedic massage doesn't really flush every single "toxin" from your system? They sure do feel good.

Some services are particularly well-suited to those with baby on board. Here are our personal picks.

Massages

The occasional rubdown might help improve blood flow and lymphatic drainage, which reduces swelling, as well as possibly improve backaches, joint pain, digestive ails, and pelvic discomfort. Shiatsu, Swedish, hot-stone, myofascial, Reiki, deep-tissue, lomi lomi, acupressure and, of course, prenatal…there's no end to the variety out there. Our fave? Watsu or "aquassage," which incorporates the smooth, relaxing strokes of Swedish massage with the gravity-defying comforts of water submersion.

Whatever you choose, be sure to ask for a masseuse familiar with pregnancy's particularities, so the necessary modifications can be made, such as lying on your side, extra pillows for support, and frequent position changes.

Bonus: If you have good health insurance, your bimonthly meeting with Manuel and his magical hands might be covered under your plan, provided he's a licensed massage therapist.

Facials

A good extraction facial can help reduce blackheads and many of the other hormonal horrors pregnancy has wrought upon your complexion, at least temporarily. If you're not a fan of all the squeezing and poking, a gentle European facial with lots of pore-opening steam and cooling toners is all pleasure and no pain.

Nails

A regular mani-pedi appointment will leave you feeling, well, polished. Sure, you could do it yourself, but it just isn't the same, now is it? Besides, after about thirty weeks, you'll be lucky if you can *see* your toes, let alone push your cuticles back.

Bonus: Salon-quality polish brands contain fewer sketchy chemicals (like phthalates and formaldehyde) than that cheap bottle of quick-dry that's been congealing in your bathroom cabinet for two years. If, however, you prefer to be completely, topically chemically-free during your pregnancy (or at least during the first trimester), a plain bubble-and-buff can be just as fabulous, and totally phthalate-free to boot!

Blowouts

That glorious mane of yours has never looked better, so why not treat it to a professional styling once in a while? A strong arm and a round brush can add volume *and* lift your mood. Now that you're extra-gorgeous, make a reservation at your favorite restaurant and have a romantic date before it's too late.

Mudwraps

Pregnant skin doesn't always glow. It can be scaly and dry and oily and itchy, all at the same time. Basting in seaweed, mud, clay, or even chocolate feels great and may help solve any epidermal enigmas. Just make sure that your body temperature stays low (turn down anything involving a heating blanket), that nothing gets wrapped too tightly, to use baby-friendly products, and to remember that you need to be able to shift positions while you marinate.

Acupuncture

Okay, so the ancient Chinese art isn't exactly a beauty treatment, but many spas and wellness centers across the country now list the service among their growing list of pseudomedical offerings. Some women hail the precise placement of tiny needles as a miracle—the only thing that helps ease morning sickness, stress, and swelling, and all without drugs. As always, tell the practitioner you're pregnant, so that certain points can be avoided.

Mock Champagne #2

Now that you're feeling a little less bitter and a little more energized, we have here for you a popular, though slightly more complicated, mock-champagne recipe. This one's designed for a larger party, but we know you'll be prepping it just for yourself and your lovey during a quiet night at home, Valentine's Day-style. Also, a great choice for baby showers.

$\frac{1}{2}$ cup sugar

$1\frac{1}{2}$ cups water

$\frac{1}{2}$ cup orange juice

2 cups cranberry juice

1 cup pineapple juice

2 (7-oz.) bottles lemon–lime soda

Using the sugar and water, create simple syrup by boiling them together in a large pot until the sugar dissolves. While the syrup cools, stir together cranberry, pineapple, and orange juices, and chill. Since you're experimenting with your own moody taste buds, slowly add soda and simple syrup to the juice mixture until you reach the right sweetness saturation point. Pour into champagne flutes and toast!

Hair Removal

When you're pregnant, you're hairy. It's a gravely serious problem, and one that warrants a more detailed examination.

Body hair may very well be the bane of your existence during pregnancy and beyond. Many previously smooth women are mortified to see their bellies suddenly become horribly hirsute (though other luckier ladies claim their leg and body hair *stops* growing). Mustaches appear seemingly overnight, rogue wiry devils emerge from moles, and toes and chins are somehow vaguely fuzzier.

The situation up top is equally precarious. We know a girl (hint: she's one of the writers of this book) whose hair turned completely white at the temples during her second pregnancy—a sign of the many frights to come. Also be aware that a few months after delivery, that luscious mane of yours, courtesy of those happy hormones which stalled the regular follicle fall-out cycle, will suddenly begin to thin. Every hair you held onto during those nine months will make a break for it: at the end of your morning shower (if you're lucky enough to get one), it will seem as if a family of small rodents drowned in the tub and then failed to get sucked down the drain.

So style and enjoy that full and fabulous head of hair while you've still got it. Though plenty of doctors say that dyeing it, perming it, or relaxing it—among the top prenatal beauty debates of all time—is fine, many women choose to wait until after the first trimester or perhaps after delivery to go crazy with chemicals. Similarly, bottle blondes might want to stick to highlights-only during their gestations, since a full head of bleach can be undeniably noxious to sensitive scalps and noses.

While the hair on your head has never looked better, it's a different story everywhere else. Unsightly bodily bristles can be banished and, quite frankly, should be. But how? One word: **waxing.** All other techniques are either too difficult, too painful, or bad for baby.

Yes, waxing will have your whiskers—and your worries—waning in no time. We recommend the full package: upper lip, underarm, belly, leg, bikini…basically, wherever you need it. And forget that myth about making things worse. A wax or a shave will *not* lead to thicker hair later. Once your pregnancy's over, your body should eventually settle back into its regular state of fuzziness.

Pregnancy and delivery present a world of woes when it comes to the bikini region in particular, since you'll have lost sight of it almost entirely by the end of your second trimester. Sure, you could go natural, but if you're planning on a nice, medicalized hospital delivery—no judgments here, the more drugs the merrier, we always say—then you should also anticipate a steady stream of doctors, nurses, medical students, and orderlies coming and going during your stay. All will check your chart, most will cop a quick feel of your cervix (though probably not the orderly, unless you ask him very nicely), and a hardy few will examine you under the unforgiving glare of a dinner plate–sized magnifying glass rimmed with 8,000-watt fluorescence. You yourself might want to watch the delivery in a mirror. All this to say…never has a bikini wax been more in order.

Since you'll want to time everything just right, being prepared is your best aesthetic. If your doc says labor is imminent, for example, wax away if you haven't done so already. Otherwise, you can expect a good grooming to last two to three weeks, so just stay smooth by keeping up with regular appointments and you should be fairly presentable, whether baby arrives early, on time, or two weeks late.

If you happen to have a crush on your obstetrician, then the storied **Brazilian** might be for you. Though the method may be pure madness, the reasoning behind the zero-hair theory is sound. Back in your mother's day, some misconceptions about cleanliness and contamination during delivery meant she was probably subjected to a full shave below the belt. Not anymore—unless you happen to be having a C-section—but the idea isn't as daft as most modern moms may think.

A good, clean waxing will leave you not only looking smooth on the big day, but feeling better during those weeks afterwards when you're experiencing what can only be described as the Period from Hell. (Sorry—we never intended to be the first to tell you about the dreaded lochia, but you may as well get used to the idea now.) Happily, by the end of your hospital experience, you'll likely be far more mellow when it comes to your intimate grooming—an unexpected side effect of those thrice-daily vaginal and hemorrhoidal inspections. But as liberating as no longer caring about such things can be, you'll feel extra comfortable knowing you're immaculately groomed.

If you're craving a Cosmo just thinking about it, better go book a massage to calm yourself down.

Belly Busters

Some spa treatments border on medical procedures—many facilities even employ dermatologists onsite these days—and can therefore be quite invasive. Whenever a service involves putting stuff directly onto your skin or into some personal crevice, inform the artist you're with child so that fetus-friendly techniques and products can be used.

A few treatments to avoid during pregnancy:

- **Tanning:** While self-tanners appear to be safe, no conclusive studies have confirmed this, so pale is the new pretty for you—particularly during the first trimester, when erring on the side of caution is your number-one job. And forget tanning beds—too hot for both your baby and your sensitive pregnancy skin.

- **Medicalized skin treatments:** The techniques used to treat the effects of aging, acne, and sun damage sometimes involve harsh products and procedures not proven safe during pregnancy. While you may be tempted to break out the big guns in the fight against wrinkles, zits, and discoloration (like chloasma—the so-called "mask" of pregnancy), rein it in. That means *no* acid peels or anything involving the following words: alpha-hydroxy (AHA), beta-hydroxy (BHA), vitamin-A, glycolic, salicylic, lactic, trichloroacetic (TCA), phenol, benzoyl-peroxide, hydroquinone, retinol, or tretinoin (Retin-A). Anything which requires a local anesthetic, like laser resurfacing, is also out.

- **Injectables:** Steer clear of Botox (paralyzing poisons and baby don't mix) and line- or lip-fillers like Restylane and collagen, as well as sclerotherapy (spider- and varicose-vein treatment via the injection of solutions).

- **Laser and chemical hair removal; bleaching:** If you dare wear short shorts, shave or wax instead and leave the chemicals and sci-fi for later. Not only are their full effects on your growing baby unknown, but your skin may be extra sensitive now.

- **Hot tubs and saunas:** Raising your body temperature

above normal may be dangerous for the baby, so stay out of the Jacuzzi. And sorry about that eucalyptus steam room, too—we know it's the real reason you joined the gym in the first place.

3. Chocolate: Better Than Sex!

There are two kinds of women in this world: those who prefer chocolate, and those who prefer sex. Most polls—and not just those conducted by the chocolate companies—suggest that the general public is pretty much split down the middle on this one. Thankfully, we're rarely forced to choose between sex and chocolate (in fact, they go together quite nicely), but during pregnancy you may find yourself settling more into one camp than the other. Happily, there's nothing preventing you from switch-hitting as you travel the rocky road to motherhood. Some days, sex will feel like the perfect way to let off some steam and have fun; on others, physical intimacy may seem like a logistical and emotional nightmare—and that's the perfect time to turn to good old Uncle Hershey for a great big hug from the inside.

For some of us, just a taste of chocolate is enough to deliver us from the doldrums and into the arms of the divine. Part of its ambrosial appeal lies in the way it dissolves on the tongue; since chocolate's melting point is slightly lower than your body temperature, tasting it becomes an active pleasure. And once it hits your system, the fireworks start immediately—your troubles begin to melt away as surely as if you'd just popped open a bottle of champagne. Best of all, not only will a square of this delectable delight deliver an instant jolt of sensory pleasure, but the buzz that follows is just as sweet.

Quite amazingly, the science is on your side if you want to draft this able ally against alcohol: numerous studies suggest that chocolate has a distinct and measurable effect on both your body and your brain. It can elevate your mood, reduce inhibitions, act as an aphrodisiac, and satisfy your oral fixations in one fell swoop. Sound familiar? Sure, it does. Only chocolate, unlike alcohol, is *all* good.

Magical Ingredients

According to painstaking research (where do we apply for *that* job?), chocolate is made up of more than three hundred distinct chemicals and compounds. Of those, the following five are the ones to thank for its bewitching buzz. Although they're only present in chocolate in very small amounts, the whole is always greater than the sum of its parts…

Hot Vanilla

Sometimes, dare we say it, you might not feel like chocolate, but still ache for that little something extra to get you in the mood. This hot drink is almost too good to be true, and discovering the sweet and sexy taste of hot vanilla is bound to get you excited....Sorry—are we going too far? Okay, we'll stop now. But take our word for it: different is good.

1 ¾ cups milk

2 oz. whipping cream

half a vanilla bean

1 ½ tsp. sugar

sprinkle of ground cinnamon, for garnish

In a heavy saucepan, combine milk, cream, vanilla bean, and sugar, and warm over low heat. When small bubbles appear around the sides of the pan, remove from heat and let sit at room temperature for fifteen to twenty minutes. Next, rewarm the mixture, whisking it briefly to redistribute the skin that forms on the surface. Remove the vanilla-bean half, scrape out the seeds with a sharp knife, and return the seeds to the milk. Pour into an eight-ounce mug and top with sprinklings of cinnamon. Drink hot. This makes enough for two servings—one for you and one for the baby.

Tryptophan

Tryptophan is an amino acid used by the brain to make serotonin, a neurotransmitter which simultaneously calms you down and lifts you up. Tryptophan is also present in turkey, and often hailed as the reason why we drift so happily off to sleep after Thanksgiving dinner.

Phenethylamine

Phenethylamine promotes the release of the neurotransmitter dopamine in the brain's pleasure centers, which means it basically revs us up like an amphetamine would. It's also responsible for chocolate's rep as an aphrodisiac, since it elevates mood, triggers euphoric feelings, dampens depression, and mimics the pleasureful effects of love (and lust). Phenethylamine levels peak during orgasm, FYI.

Theobromine

Theobromine is similar to its chemical cousin caffeine in that it has a mood-elevating effect. But unlike the quick kick of caff, which increases stress in the brain, theobromine is far gentler a lover. Theobromine, by the way, is what makes chocolate dangerous for dogs and cats, whose bodies metabolize it far slower than ours do. If you've ever had to induce Fifi into bringing up that bag of Kisses she got into, you know what we're talking about. But one woman's poison is another one's pleasure—especially if that woman happens to be pregnant—so just keep the goods on the top shelf from now on.

Anandamide
Anandamide is one of the so-called cannabinoid neurotransmitters, and you can probably guess what that means—that chocolate and being stoned are somehow intertwined. You're right: anandamide stimulates the exact same brain receptors that the cannabis in marijuana and hashish do, mimicking their effects quite nicely in large enough amounts. Now you can say "I didn't inhale" with pride and still get happy and be healthy.

Endorphins
Like exercise, laughter, and sex, sugary foods release endorphins (specifically, beta-endorphins), which make you feel calm, happy, and reduce feelings of pain in the brain. That endorphin rush is why heroin addicts also crave sweets, and it's also why a hungry, chocolate-yearning, alcohol-deprived pregnant woman could kick a junkie's ass in a fight for an Almond Joy any day of the week.

To sum up, any prenatal fondness for fondant is probably worth indulging. If you want to get the most out of its intoxicating effects, visit the dark side: while milk chocolate's creamier qualities may appeal to your palate, the darker version contains higher concentrations of the good stuff, not to mention less fat and less sugar.

Chocolate Maternitini

For those days when chocolate is better than sex—and there will be many—this is a nice way to settle into an after-dinner treat. It will get your PEAs a-poppin'—that's short for phenethylamine, the famous "love-chemical" of chocolate. As you're pouring your third, remind your partner that a few of these will certainly make for a more amorous mood...

Ice

Instant hot-chocolate powder

2 oz. of melted chocolate (or chocolate syrup, if that's easier)

1 oz. half-and-half

$1/4$ teaspoon vanilla extract, optional

Coat the rim of a martini glass with hot-chocolate powder. Refrigerate glass. Mix ingredients together with ice in a cocktail shaker. Strain carefully into your chilled martini glass.

Belly Busters

Before you go completely cuckoo for cocoa puffs, remember that chocolate does contain a little bit of **caffeine**. An average bar boasts way less than a cup if joe, but if you have a caffeine allergy or are ingesting seriously massive amounts of dark chocolate, which has slightly higher caffeine concentrations, you might start to feel a little jittery. While most health care professionals agree that even the caff contained in a daily latte or two is fine for your fetus, too much of anything can be a bad thing, so try and keep it in control. The term chocoholic may be more than a cute way to describe your romance with Mars bars. Believe it or not, some studies suggest that chocolate has a similar **addictive quality** to that of alcohol. All in all, though, this confection is perfection if you're looking for a temporary stand-in for spirits for the next nine months. Oh, and as we mentioned earlier, stay away from ingesting multiple boxes of liqueur-filled chocolate in a single sitting. You're not fooling anyone.

And of course, no discussion about chocolate would be complete without its attending evil, **weight gain**…but we don't really want to go there, do we? Suffice it to say that only you, your obstetrician, and your tailor know how much weight gain is right for you, and only you know how comfortable you feel exceeding that limit.

4. Sex: Better Than Chocolate!

For some lucky women, pregnancy sex is the best of their lives. For others, chocolate still takes the cake, and might continue to do so until that baby bump is away at summer camp, or at least visiting the in-laws for a sleepover. But if you keep an open mind to all the glorious possibilities of prenatal nookie, you too might be drunk with love before you know it.

We can't promise it's always going to be easy, because let's face it—self-image issues, paralyzing exhaustion, physical ails, and psychological angst are pretty much anathema to feeling randy. The good news? Getting in the mood may be the biggest obstacle you face in your quest for excellent pregnancy sex, but knowing the Nine Reasons Pregnant Sex Rocks and following our Nine Steps to Nine Months of Super Sex, both on the following pages, will help you realize it's more than worth it.

If you're struggling with morning sickness, take heart: the second trimester is just around the corner, and they don't call it the "Honeymoon Phase" for nothing. Weeks thirteen through twenty-eight will likely find you feeling way less sick, less tired, and still not too large to be physically uncomfortable—the perfect time to go for a roll in the hay. Once the third trimester rears its ugly head, the combination of your tremendous girth, nervous anticipation, and various gestational ills might get in the way of your flirtatious spirit once again, which is why we recommend you get busy now while the getting's still good.

Overall, just take it day by day and remain positive about sex. No matter what stage of pregnancy you're in, your mood and your body will dictate your level of lustiness, so stay in tune with yourself and get ready to go at a moment's notice.

Nine Reasons Pregnant Sex Rocks

Sex during pregnancy is extra-fun for oh so many reasons. Here are nine, just in case you need a little extra encouragement to inspire you…

1. Increased Blood Volume: By the time you deliver that baby, you will be carrying up to 50 percent more blood than usual. And that means *everywhere,* girlfriend. All this engorgement and throbbing bodes quite well for your love life.

2. Stress Relief: It's hard to worry about what color to paint the nursery or that nasty rival at work when you're having the best sex ever.

3. Better Orgasms: Mysterious but true—some women are only orgasmic during pregnancy; others are multiorgasmic for the first time. Don't overthink it. Just do it.

4. Super Sleep: Instead of tossing and turning for hours, you'll drift off gently into dreamland from the warm, fuzzy haze of post-coital bliss…at least until you wake up an hour later to pee.

5. No More Birth Control: Nice not to have to worry about it for a change, isn't it?

6. Improved Intimacy: Sex is an ideal way to stay connected with your partner. Plus, if you foster a healthy love life during your pregnancy, the deposits you make now can be drawn on during the long dry months ahead. Or, it'll backfire and your partner will have trouble going cold turkey after the birth and turn into a masturbating fiend. Oh, well—at least you're having fun in the meantime.

7. Fun with Positions: When you're almost too big to move and playing cowgirl is out, think outside the box. Don't be shy—you're about to have a child with this person, and any shred of modesty you currently retain will be obliterated during the delivery anyway. Pregnancy is also the perfect time to take up Tantric sex, the anti-quickie. If you can't get Sting to give you some pointers, pick up a how-to book and go gently into that good night together. Also invest in a copy of the Kama Sutra to open your eyes to the possibilities. After all, necessity is the mother of invention. And the mother needs sex. *Now.*

8. Gets the Show on the Road: Are your forty weeks up? Your health care professional might encourage you to have sex in the hopes of bringing on labor. At the very least, it can't hurt. (Note: If you've already lost your mucus plug, which prevents bacteria from passing through the cervix, no nookie for you.) Not quite there yet? We know what you're thinking, dear, but don't worry: though some studies suggest that sex—in particular, the uterine-contracting effects of the female orgasm, or possibly even the prostaglandin in semen—might help labor along late in the game, there's no, um, hard evidence to suggest that lovemaking during a normal, healthy pregnancy will cause you to go into labor prematurely.

9. Secret Bonus: Get your partner drunk to put him in the mood, and then enjoy a little taste of heaven with a French kiss. That hint of hooch on his breath will make you drunk, too—with *love*.

Nine Steps to Nine Months of Super Sex

To increase your chances of enjoying a great sex life while you're pregnant, employ the following rules of engagement and get busy!

1. Keep the Lines of Communication Open: The healthier your relationship is and the fewer things left unsaid the hotter your love life will be. Address any concerns immediately, whether they be about sex or the phone bill.

2. Listen to Your Body: If you're tired at night, why not make a romantic lunch date instead? Take advantage of those days when you feel good and get going.

3. Book It: Scheduling may not sound romantic, but that little heart on the calendar for next Friday night will give you something to look forward to. Makes it more likely to actually happen, too.

4. Stay Fit, Eat Well: The better you feel physically the more likely you'll be to want to see if that gorgeous new glow of yours will rub off on your significant other.

5. Instigate Things: If you're used to being pursued, try on the hunter's hat for a change. Your partner may be a little more hesitant than usual these days (for too many reasons to count), and now's not the time for you to, um, drop the ball.

6. Be Brave: Missionary, shmissionary. Now's when you both need to get creative in the sack, for both necessity's sake and just for the fun of it.

7. Fool Around: You don't have to hit a home run every time—there are three other bases worth stealing. When it comes to pregnancy and sex, you score just by playing the game.

8. Know You're Gorgeous: Not to be sappy or trite, but pregnancy really is a beautiful state of being. Though it may *feel* like crap sometimes, never will your body be more perfect that it is during your gestation, when its beguiling balance of form and function becomes a testament to the fundamental coolness of the entire reproductive process. Don't just tell yourself you look good—*believe* it.

9. Put Yourself in His Shoes: Remember, it's been all about you lately. Keep your partner's needs in mind, and let him know you're still attracted to him, that you understand what he's going through, too. Empathy breeds intimacy, in the bedroom and out.

We like to think that the myriad blessings of pregnancy

sex are your body's way of saying thanks, a kind of gentle payback for everything it's been putting you through since that little plus sign showed up on the HPT. And because sex *after* baby arrives is likely to be, well, not quite as good—at least for the first few months—you may as well take advantage of things now. There's no reason why you guys shouldn't be one of the lucky couples who enjoys this time to the fullest.

Belly Busters

- Alas, sometimes sex should be avoided during pregnancy for **health reasons**. If you've had premature contractions, pain, spotting, a loss of your mucus plug, or an incompetent cervix; if you're carrying multiples; or if you're on bed rest or pelvic rest for any reason, you will probably be advised to lay off getting laid at some point. It sucks, we know, but like abstaining from alcohol, saying no to sex is absolutely necessary if it endangers anyone.

- There is also a debate raging about **nipple stimulation** and its relationship to premature labor. Nipple stimulation, like orgasm, does release oxytocin, the hormone that causes contractions, so if you have a history of late-term miscarriage or preterm labor, or want to err on the side of caution, avoid it.

- Nervous partners can easily be put at ease if you lay

a little education their way. Any **fears about hurting the baby** will quickly be quelled by a reassuring conversation with your doctor or midwife during your next appointment. Remember, too, that flattery will get you everywhere; a little precoital exposition—something along the lines of, "You're *so* well-endowed, darling…isn't it amazing how my cervix is designed to completely protect the baby during intercourse?!"—will not only get him in the mood, but remind him that everything's going to be just fine.

- If your significant other seems disinterested, **attraction** might be the issue. The best approach to take here is a gradual one. If your partner hasn't seen your naked belly for six months and you suddenly drop your robe to reveal that new and more bountifully sized Agent Provocateur push-up, your grotesquely distended abdomen might prove a little distracting. Instead, make sure to involve him in your blossoming physique from the very beginning. Seeing you change slowly over time is not only less likely to terrify him, but fooling around as often as you can early on will make things way less weird later.

GETTING A SOCIAL LIFE:

Birthdays, Barbecues, and Barflies, Oh My!

"I'm sick of being the designated driver—why can't they all just take a bloody cab?"

—*Jenny B., 23, Portland, OR*

At home, where *you* control the environment, it's way easier to keep things calm, cool, and collected in your quest to keep the spirits at bay. But step out your front door and in an instant, the entire universe is conspiring against you, from four-story-high Absolut ads around every corner to those free wine cooler samples at your local Costco. Add your usual social life into the mix and your old pal alcohol suddenly seems more like a stalker. Or, to seriously misquote Samuel Taylor Coleridge, there's firewater, firewater everywhere, but not a drop to drink.

Yes, maintaining a decent social life among the carefree, non-gestating masses can be a challenge, to say the least. Getting through the best parties of the year without your favorite cocktail is not going to be easy, and meeting the girls for "drinks" after work certainly won't be the same as it used to. That said, there's no need to become a shut-in for the next nine months. If you're willing to start thinking about things in a new light, there are still plenty of happy birthdays ahead and fun to be had.

Just like old times…sort of. These poolside favorites or Super Bowl Sunday substitutes will keep you feeling like you're still in the mix. Even friends who aren't on the wagon will be begging you to mix one up for them, too.

Virgin Margarita

We hated giving up this summertime classic during our pregnancies, when just seeing those salt-rimmed margarita glasses made us pant like Pavlov's dogs. In that spirit, we've modified the Official Drink of Summer with that bun in your oven in mind. We highly recommend our version for all those outdoor summer events: barbecues, beach days, and pool parties. As always, blended with ice is twice as nice.

Ice

1 ½ oz. sour mix

½ oz. lime juice

½ oz. orange juice

Lime wedges, for garnish

Pour ingredients (minus the lime wedges) into a cocktail shaker. Shake and pour into a rocks glass or a margarita glass. Add more ice if needed. Our highly recommended alternative is to blend in a blender with ice. Garnish with a wedge of lime.

Variation: If you're not in a do-it-yourself mood, lemon and/or lime margarita mix works just as well. Frozen or on the rocks, it's up to you; just make sure you garnish with a lime and squeeze the juice into the drink. You almost won't miss the tequila. (Yeah, right.)

Party On

We bet you never realized how pro-alcohol the world was until you became part of the prohibition. The problem, of course, is that you're still invited to the party.

Whereas before you became pregnant, those days off couldn't come fast enough, now it seems like your calendar's just one long sangria-soaked weekend after another. Starting with New Year's Eve, there's a government-sanctioned reason to drink virtually every month until Christmas, not counting all the birthdays, bachelorette parties, christenings, clambakes, retirements, engagements, housewarmings, and weddings in between. Even an 11 a.m. bris on a Tuesday is stacked to the rafters with Manishevitz. So where exactly does this leave you?

As the lucky lady stockpiling nine months' worth of favors, that's where!

Without further ado, here's how to turn the traditionally tiresome trappings of teetotaling into terrific opportunities for fun and profit.

Keep the Meter Running

Under normal circumstances, being the designated driver is annoying—a burden undertaken on a rotating basis and then only in the certain absence of cabs and/or public transportation. When you're in a family way, however, you'd do well to relish the task of taxi driver. You see, it's all about the payback. Nine months of door-to-door service is unlikely to be forgotten, no matter how drunk your fares are.

Virgin Mai Tai

This drink—which originated in California in the 1940s and takes its name from the Tahitian word for good—will make you wish you were reliving that special vacay to "anywhere but here" right about now. We wish you warm and relaxing, alcohol-laced honeymoon memories as you sip one of these in your backyard.

Ice

4 oz. pineapple juice

2 oz. orange juice

2 oz. club soda

1 tbsp. cream of coconut

1 tbsp. grenadine

Cherries, for garnish

Pour ingredients into a cocktail shaker and shake. Pour into a collins glass, adding additional ice if necessary, and garnish with a cherry and an umbrella.

Help the Drunk Girl

Just because you're not living in the sorority house anymore doesn't mean your friends are above the obnoxiousness of collegial carousing, as you probably know all too well already. Every once in a while, somebody gets dumped or declares bankruptcy and suddenly you're in Vegas, two blocks off the Strip and twenty miles from morality, with the former Miss Goody Two-Shoes herself slung across the bar for body shots. Your new role as den mother means you get to be the one who makes sure things don't get *too* out of control, and later, maybe hold her hair back while she's doubled over the bowl—provided your own sensitive tummy can handle it, of course. A few months down the line, when you score last-minute concert tickets and desperately need a baby-sitter for your colicky kid, guess who's getting the call?

Extract Secrets and Break Bad News

Alcohol's reputation as a truth-serum is indeed well-founded, and drunk people are an untapped resource. If you're looking for the scoop, now's the time to get it. For example, you might want to use this chance to ask for personal favors if you're around friends and family, or hustle some professional advice or deadline extensions if it's a work function. Booze-soaked social events also afford an excellent opportunity to break bad news, as in "Sorry, Aunt Bea, but Fred and I won't be able to come to Fifi's obedience-school graduation party. Can I get you another mimosa?"

Two by Abacus Restaurant, Dallas, TX

Terry Kranz of Abacus—one of the top restaurants in Dallas—suggested these fantastic mocktails for when your mojito has lost its mojo and your cran seems kind of bland. Or, if you're in the neighborhood, go have Terry mix one up for you personally at 4511 McKinney Avenue, Dallas, TX, 75205.

Spring Mint

Ice

2 oz. Rose's Lime Juice

2 oz. simple syrup

6 sprigs fresh mint

Club soda, to fill

Lime wedges, for garnish

Take a martini shaker and add mint, lime juice, and syrup. Fill the shaker halfway with ice. Cap and shake so that the mint is broken into little pieces, pour into a collins glass, then fill the rest with soda. Garnish with lime.

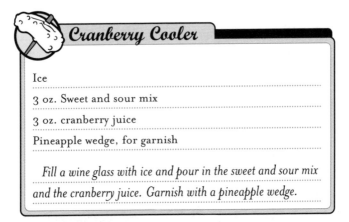

Cranberry Cooler

Ice

3 oz. Sweet and sour mix

3 oz. cranberry juice

Pineapple wedge, for garnish

Fill a wine glass with ice and pour in the sweet and sour mix and the cranberry juice. Garnish with a pineapple wedge.

Play Bartender

If you can hack it, offer to man the bar. There's plenty of truth in the old adage, "Keep your friends close, and your enemies closer," and sometimes simply participating in the rituals surrounding your old pal alcohol and its preparation will be enough to make you feel like you're still living it up, instead of drying out on the sidelines.

Unexpected Bonus: You'll also be able to mix your own mocktails and eat as many maraschino cherries and olives as you want.

Martyr Yourself for the Cause, Then Use the Baby as an Excuse

Though you may not really feel like it, accept the invitation and show your host or hostess you appreciate his or her hospitality. Later, if you're having a crappy time, just play the pregnant card and go home. Nobody would dare question your commitment to maintaining normalcy once you've made an appearance and shown a sincere attempt to be part of the fun. If anyone nasty does throw a sideways glance your way, toss in some labored breathing and extra-pathetic wobbly walking for emphasis. Your braveness in the face of physical pain and abstinence from alcohol will garner much sympathy and appreciation—and confirm your status as a woman of character.

Unexpected Bonus: The secret upside of suffering through parties and social outings stone-cold sober? When you begin to notice how idiotic drunk people really are, it may even turn you off alcohol—at least until you're allowed to become one the idiots again.

Two Frozen Poolside Classics

These two drinks are thick as thieves, hanging out on poolside drink menus like partners in crime, which is why we're listing them together. Enjoy these virgin versions liberally on a hot day as a tasty way to prevent dehydration. And here's an idea: combine half a colada with half a daiquiri to create the Arnold Palmer of frozen drinks. Bonus: if you hang out in the sun and fresh air long enough, you're bound to feel a little drunk. (Just don't forget to drink lots and slather on that sunscreen!)

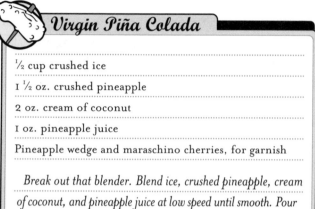

Virgin Piña Colada

½ cup crushed ice

1 ½ oz. crushed pineapple

2 oz. cream of coconut

1 oz. pineapple juice

Pineapple wedge and maraschino cherries, for garnish

Break out that blender. Blend ice, crushed pineapple, cream of coconut, and pineapple juice at low speed until smooth. Pour into a collins glass. Garnish with a pineapple wedge and a cherry.

Virgin Strawberry Daiquiri

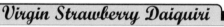

½ cup crushed ice

1 oz. fresh lime juice (about 1 lime)

3 oz. fresh strawberries (or frozen sliced strawberries in syrup)

1 tsp. sugar, or to taste

Whole strawberries and orange slices, for garnish

In a blender, combine ice, lime juice, strawberries, and sugar, and blend on low speed until smooth. Pour into chilled daiquiri glass. Garnish with a whole strawberry and an orange slice.

What to Do Instead

From time to time, you may feel that being around all that drinking is simply not going to work for you, though you still dread the thought of being a party pooper. Instead, why not recruit a few friends or loved ones and enjoy something a little different once in a while?

National Sobriety Day

If you're looking for a holiday without alcohol, this is the premier party of the year. National Sobriety Day has been recognized by various states as falling on December 11—the day Alcoholics Anonymous founder Bill Wilson stopped drinking—though sometimes it takes place earlier in the fall. Local municipalities and groups throughout the country celebrate the sober lifestyle by organizing various events and booze-free fun and games for the public. Visit www.nationalsobrietyday.com for details.

Kids' Stuff

We know—you're about to head down this road for real in a few months' time, but it wouldn't hurt you to try life on the other side. Pack a picnic and head out to family day in your local park, take in the circus or a parade, or go to the zoo. The fresh air will do you good, and the alcoholic refreshments should be at a minimum.

Culture Club

Hmm…how to enjoy a nice weekend afternoon, *without* drinking or being forced to be around people who are? Try foreign films, Shakespeare in the park, local museums, antique hunting, flea markets, musical concerts, or poetry readings. Basically, we recommend anything that gets you out of the house without turning you into a souse. Even if the activity in question is outside your normal comfort zone, give it a shot—you never know, you might like it! (St. Patrick's Day festivities don't count, by the way.)

Charity Village

Walkathons, fund-raisers, and philanthropic functions of all kinds are an excellent way to get out there and have fun, plus they're chock-full of a major value-added benefit—doing some good. The summer is virtually packed with weekend events in local parks and venues where alcohol will rarely rear its ugly head, though you should be able to count on lots of ice cream stands and other caloric crowd-pleasers to stand in. During colder months, splurge on gala tickets benefiting the museum, ballet, or hospital. Local libraries, schools, and community centers also offer plenty of opportunities to get involved. Or get back to basics with some one-on-one fun and be a Big Sister to a kid who could use a friend.

Religious Events

Whether you regularly attend church, synagogue, or mosque, your spiritual community can be a superb source of support during these trying times. Many social shindigs planned by religious institutions are alcohol-free, and though they may not be as wild as your brother-in-law's annual Fourth of July Super Beer Blowout, you're less likely to end up feeling left out. And you can tell your partner to wipe that look off his face—his new role in life is to support you every sober step of the way.

Brown Pigskin

Okay, fall has fallen and it's finally football season, but your craving for a cold brewski is suddenly offside. First, put down the beer—you're way better off with piles of potato chips smothered in French onion dip. Second, send your partner into the kitchen to whip you up one of these, which will keep you satisfied as you settle into the second quarter. GO TEAM!

Ice

5 oz. apple cider

2 ½ oz. ginger beer

Fill highball glass with ice, then gently pour in the cider and ginger beer. Stir.

Raising the Bar

Let's face it—no matter how hard they try, most of your friends simply don't care about your burgeoning bump and newly delicate sensibilities as much as you do, and therefore probably aren't willing to relocate any upcoming bachelorette parties to the church basement. Nor is taking that potential client you've been trying to land for drinks at Chuck E. Cheese likely to go over well. But just because you're with child doesn't mean that bars, like parties, are suddenly off-limits. And it's a good thing, too, since a great many of us spend plenty of time in drinking establishments, enjoying special events, professional shmoozing, and personal socializing alike.

Though bars and clubs present a new slew of problems for pregnant you, some simple planning can ensure you don't get left out in the cold.

Gregg's Greatest Hits
by Gregg Horan of Luxbar and Gibsons

Well, we love our friend Gregg Horan of Chicago's Luxbar and the legendary Gibsons Steakhouse. When we asked for a few of his faves for a nonalcoholic night out, here's what he offered. They may not be of the "mix-it-yourself" variety for everyone, but write 'em down, tear 'em out, and challenge your local bartender to make 'em as well as Gregg can. (If you're in town, go see him yourself at Gibsons, 1028 North Rush Street, Chicago, IL, 60611. Luxbar is at 118 East Bellevue, Chicago, IL, 60611.)

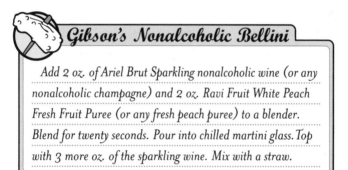

Luxbar Strawberry Sling

Muddle two large strawberries in a collins glass

Add ice

Add 1 ½ oz. simple syrup

Add 2 oz. fresh lemon juice

Add 2 oz. water

Shake vigorously in a martini shaker. Return to collins glass, top with club soda, and garnish with a strawberry.

Gibson's Nonalcoholic Bellini

Add 2 oz. of Ariel Brut Sparkling nonalcoholic wine (or any nonalcoholic champagne) and 2 oz. Ravi Fruit White Peach Fresh Fruit Puree (or any fresh peach puree) to a blender. Blend for twenty seconds. Pour into chilled martini glass. Top with 3 more oz. of the sparkling wine. Mix with a straw.

Making Your Way through the Minefield

Since the widely adopted bans on smoking have come into effect in most states, bars and clubs are now far more fetus-friendly than they used to be. But despite the relatively fresh air, plenty of unexpected dangers remain lurking in the lamplight.

Here's how to tackle the challenges head-on, stand your ground, and still have fun.

Mile-High Stools

Taking a tumble from on high can bruise not only your belly, but your ego, too. As your bump grows, your weight will become less evenly distributed, so when considering where to plant yourself for the evening, the lower your center of gravity the more stable you'll be. Though sitting right at the bar makes for much merriment, Humpty Dumpty, we're sure your companions won't mind if you move it to a table instead.

Pick-Up Artists

Remember that from the waist up, you probably still look like fair game, so if your belly is below table level, don't be too outraged if some well-meaning Romeo chats you up in the hopes of getting your number. If you're already showing, smile demurely, stand up, and flash a bit of bump— seeing the look on his face makes for great sport. If you're feeling extra playful (or if you found the fellow offensive to begin with), pretend like you expect him not to care and hint that you're in the market for a new daddy for baby.

If you still have abs of steel, happen to be well-camouflaged, or don't feel like engaging the opposite sex on any level, an ounce of prevention is worth a pound of cure: wearing a wedding ring (whether you're married or not) and showing it off will nine times out of ten keep a prospective suitor at bay. Unless, of course, he's a drunken idiot...

Drunken Idiots

Liquor can turn even the mildest-mannered of men into leering Lotharios. If some loser gets up in your grill, don't be afraid to react fast. Employ your friends' help to get rid of him, or let a bartender or bouncer know you don't appreciate this particular patron. Most establishments have a strict no-harassment policy, and proprietors empower their staff with the right to refuse service, threaten expulsion, or actually kick out on their butt any person deemed offensive or threatening to the other customers. In extreme cases, when you need to make a point, and fast, a drink in the face or a well-placed knee will let that loser know Mama Bear means business when it comes to protecting her cub. If the guy keeps coming at you, other people will surely step in to make sure he gets what's coming to him.

Invasions of Personal Space

For many of us, claustrophobia and germophobia are common pregnancy symptoms, and crowded public places can try our patience to the max. To counteract people problems in bars and clubs, survey the joint the second you walk in—bathrooms, emergency exits, coatrooms, dance-floor placement, and bar location all play a role in determining traffic flow and potential bottlenecks, and must be carefully considered when choosing a spot to sit. What you want to do is create a nice, secure, open perimeter of space around yourself at all times, with plenty of room to breathe and shift positions, both while seated and while on the move. If at any time the bar becomes simply too crowded for you to be comfortable, we highly advise you hightail it out of there. Avoiding accidental injury is far more important than maintaining your pre-pregnancy urban awesomeness, at least for now.

If you're feeling frazzled, let your friends get your drinks for you, or wait for the waitress to come around. When you do decide to head out into the fray—whether you're on the way to the loo or the dance floor—avail yourself of any and all tactical maneuvers you can think of to ensure your continued comfort and safety. Being on defense at all times will help defuse any potential problems before they arise. A vigilant chaperone and some subtly placed knees, elbows, and heels will keep you and your belly from being accidentally knocked into or bumped around.

Dance-Floor Safety

Many normal social niceties are suspended in the tight spaces of the dance floor and/or concert hall. If you do plan to bust a move, keep the Manolos in the closet and opt instead for flats, kitten heels, or wedges; you'll need to be super-stable to stay safe and have fun. Again, prioritize your need for personal space and enlist the help of friends to form a protective barrier between you and the sweaty masses. If you feel faint or dizzy at any time, retreat—being trampled is contraindicated to pregnancy. Rest and refuel before heading back out there. And we don't need to tell you to leave the rough stuff, like mosh pits and crowd-surfing, to the kiddies while you're with child.

Contending with Clueless Bartenders

Not everybody can mix a decent mocktail, especially at pubs and other more common drinking establishments. For your part, you can adjust your expectations to suit the situation—say, you're at the sports bar during playoffs or accompanying your significant other to his favorite brew-and-knockwurst tent at Oktoberfest—and stick to juices or sodas. If, however, you suspect an ample assortment of imported grenadines and a 150-horsepower blender behind the bar, step right up. Look that mixologist square in the eye and ask for what you want. Speak loudly and clearly over the din, or else be prepared to get a Sex on the Beach when you requested a Virgin Georgia with Peach.

Alas, you may occasionally encounter that all-too-familiar enemy of an inspired cocktail: the Warm Body behind the Bar. This unimaginative sort has a recipe repertoire of about four drinks, and can't mix his or her way out of a paper bag. When you encounter that clue-less stare, or fear your request is about to be mangled, explicit instructions are in order.

At the end of this book, you'll find some cut-out squares printed with a few simple yet smashing mocktail recipes capable of being produced behind any reasonably well-stocked bar. Or, you can make your own to pass out—just scribble your favorite formula on the back of some of your business cards and keep them in your wallet for handy access. Who knows? You might even make a few contacts along the way.

Sweet Tart

Put on your party shoes (since they're the only things left that still fit you—probably) and head out to the bar with the recipe for this tart concoction tucked into your purse (since it's the only thing left that still fits you—definitely). The Sweet Tart has "shooter" written all over it, and remember: the lemonade in this puppy will sting if you need to throw a drink in someone's face. Now, pucker up!

Ice

2 oz. cranberry juice

2 oz. ginger ale

2 oz. lemonade

Mix ingredients in a cocktail shaker with ice and strain into a shooter glass. Alternately, it also looks pretty on ice in a wine glass. If you find it too tart, simply cut back on the lemonade. (As with all our recipes, tweak to your taste.)

Dealing with Bothersome Bladders

Frequent urination in frequently disgusting situations is a problem you're likely to experience in your quest to maintain a normal social life. From the moment you pee on that stick, your bladder will betray you for, well, the rest of your life. (If you're lucky, things will improve slightly in the months after delivery). And when you're drinking—even if it's without the added diuretic effects of alcohol—you're sure to be visiting the ladies' room more often than normal.

The following four strategies will help you master common bathroom blunders while baby's on board.

1. Say Hello to Hand Sanitizer: Pregnancy is a great time to explore your inner germophobe, and public watering holes will give you ample opportunity to disinfect. Quick-drying liquid disinfectant comes in convenient travel sizes and we advise you invest in a multipack. Filthy locks and door handles, as well as empty soap and towel dispensers, will have you singing its praises in no time.

2. Carry Your Own Covers: It may be a little, um, anal, but what would you prefer—that your blessed backside make actual contact with some squalid seat and possibly pick up public pubes or pee or worse? The drugstore sells packages of portable covers. Avail yourself of them every time you've got to go. If you don't have a cover handy, make one out of toilet paper. None left? Change stalls or squat above the seat.

3. Keep the Kleenex Handy: No TP? No problem. Remember to pack a pack before you leave the house. Your purse should be virtually bursting with kitteny softness at all times.

4. For Heaven's Sake, Do Those Lunges!: The Holy Grail of lavatory mastery for the pregnant woman with a penchant for public places is strong hamstrings and glutes. If you can squat over the seat through your fortieth week, you can conquer the world.

Shot in the Pot

In the mood for something that hurts? Since a shot of Jack is obviously out of the question, try this one on for size when you need to feel your throat burn. Warning: this is not for the morning-sick or the faint-of-heart. Your eyes will water, your chest will seize, and you may temporarily lose your vision. On the upside, if you're a week or two overdue and looking for a way to induce labor, this one's for you.

½ oz. ginger ale, chilled

½ oz. Tabasco sauce

Combine ingredients in shot glass and shoot.

chapter

6

SOBRIETY SUPPORT:

The New Twelve Steps and How to Take Them

"Some days, it's hard to keep my eye on the prize when my mind is trying a vodka martini on for size. How do I stay focused when I feel so frazzled?"

—*Wendy C., 29, Toronto, ON*

Creating an environment of support—especially within your own home and social circle—will pave the way to success for every Newly Non-Drinking Girl. Surrounding yourself with understanding and sympathetic people, maintaining a positive internal dialogue, and focusing on alternative methods of stress relief is usually more than enough ammunition to keep that cocktail-loving little devil off your shoulder for these nine long months. Sometimes, though, even the best-laid plans can fall by the wayside if you're having a tough day.

Yes, that pregnant glow can quickly lose its luster when things don't go exactly as planned. Wait…did you believe that just because a bun happens to be baking in your oven that you'd be as blissful as Betty Crocker every waking moment? Quite the opposite, actually—you're in the middle of what many women cite as the most stressful time of their lives. The combination of physical, emotional, professional, and financial pressures you face every single day would be enough to bring most men to their knees. *This* is the real labor of pregnancy, and delivery doesn't exactly solve the problem, if you catch our drift. So give yourself permission to be blue; no woman, no matter how saintly, is completely immune to the ups and downs of the daily grind.

And things can quickly go from bad to worse when life throws you a curveball. If you've just been fired, lost a loved one, had a fight with your partner, are on the brink of bankruptcy, or simply feel like you're spiraling out-of-control, the temptation to turn to old friends like Jack Daniels, Jim Beam, Johnnie Walker, and Jose Cuervo can be stronger than ever.

Welcome to the Danger Zone.

Don't worry, you can admit it—you're among friends here, and we promise not to tell. We understand exactly what you're going through because we've been there...*and* come back from the brink without a drink. The key is to acknowledge your craving in order to be able to conquer it. (Denial ain't just a river in Egypt; it's also the number-one enemy you'll face in the fight against your own mind and all its liquor-soaked old habits.)

So go on and get comfortable, because you may be here a while. This chapter and the next—"Professional Help: Where to Turn When You Really Can't Go It Alone"—are your best sources for information, support, and that extra little bit of inspiration to get you over the hump and get your mind back on that bump.

The concoctions in this chapter were sent to us by various Pregnant Pause initiatives—community-based events (often hosted by bars) designed to make sobriety fun and appealing for mothers-to-be, and increase public awareness about the dangers of alcohol-exposed pregnancies.

Peppermint Pacifier

From the New Jersey Coalition for Prevention of Developmental Disabilities

Ice

$\frac{1}{2}$ oz. peppermint syrup

1 $\frac{1}{2}$ oz. chocolate syrup

2 $\frac{1}{2}$ oz. 2% milk

Whipped cream, for topping

Place all the ingredients in a blender and blend until smooth.
Serve in a large mug and garnish with whipped cream.

Twelve Sober Steps for Nine Long Months

With expediency in mind, we've condensed all of our research and experience into our very own simple-to-follow Twelve-Step Program. Not only should you welcome it as your new way of life for the next nine months, but it can also help you through any tough moments that may arise on a case-by-case basis. Consider the items "crib notes" (sorry, we couldn't resist), and turn to them as often as you need to for a sober second thought whenever temptation strikes. Put a copy of the list in your wallet, stick it on your fridge, turn it into your screensaver at work…whatever it takes, wherever life takes you.

(Please keep in mind that our little program was designed with the light to moderate drinker in mind.

For anyone out there in need of extra help, working the original Twelve Steps of Alcoholics Anonymous or following another substance-abuse recovery program may be in order, but more on that in Chapter 7.)

So without further ado, let us introduce our Twelve Sober Steps for Nine Long Months…

1. Keep a "Kosher" Home

Removing all temptation from your living space is an important precaution to take for those who feel weak-willed from time to time. Seeing your husband's bottle of Stoli in the freezer as you reach for a popsicle, or watching the sunlight glint seductively off that gorgeous crystal decanter on your dining-room sideboard may be a bit much to handle. If so, you need to do some serious spring cleaning. When there's nothing in your bar but some coasters, a half-empty shaker of celery salt, and a few bottles of tonic water, what might have been a momentary lapse in judgment will remain as harmless as a bottle of formula. So put on your beer goggles, explore the house, and edit out anything even remotely tantalizing. After all, a short stroll to the kitchen to grab a cold brewski is a whole lot easier than having to schlep your ass down to the 7-Eleven to get one.

2. Become Alcohol-Aware

Learn why exactly it is that booze and babies don't mix, and you'll find your cravings are powerless against your newfound knowledge. Spend a few hours on the Internet doing some research of your own. Read all those scary studies, if you must. Then, to banish any chance of bad behavior, get into the habit of frequently reminding yourself why that pretty blue martini just isn't worth it.

3. Practice Aversion Therapy

When a nice, cool Long Island Iced Tea would really hit the spot, fill up on a big, tall glass of bad memories instead. Crack open a bottle of Crème de Menthe and take a deep whiff: suddenly, it's 1989 and you're throwing your guts up behind the Bowl-O-Drome. We defy you to have even a *regular* iced tea after that. Yes, every Drinking Girl has at least one beverage that will bring her back to a time, place, or position she'd rather forget. Remember?

Allmom Joy

by the New Jersey Coalition for Prevention of Developmental Disabilities

Ice (1 scoop)

3 oz. 2% milk

¾ oz. almond syrup

¾ oz. coconut syrup or cream of coconut

Whipped cream, for topping

Place all ingredients in a blender and blend until smooth. Serve in a large goblet or wine glass, and garnish with whipped cream.

4. Plan Ahead to Keep Your Head

Keeping a pack of gum in your purse just won't cut it when it comes to quelling a real, alcohol-craving emergency. Know what your weaknesses are—whether they be socially inspired, stress-induced, or impulse-related—and figure out how you'll handle it when the urge to indulge strikes. If you're sure there's no possible way you'll make it through your annual Oktoberfest blowout with the girls without a pint, play sick and rent *Father of The Bride II* instead. Can't fly without fear? Leave the mini-bottles on board and take the train, or else invest in a few sessions of flight therapy.

5. Use Mind Control

Thinking about drinking? Don't indulge that naughty internal dialogue for a single minute—just get busy thinking about something else. Let's say you're at the bar with a few friends. Your favorite cocktails are two-for-one. You're not showing yet, and nobody even knows you're pregnant, for heaven's sake! It's so easy to tell yourself, *One teeny-weeny tequila couldn't hurt at this stage…*

STOP!

Do not—we repeat, *do not*—bother trying to justify it. Do not even allow yourself to entertain the notion for a nanosecond. You just pull yourself up by the sandal straps and tell that liquor-loving little voice inside your head to shut up and think about baseball instead. Or shoes. Or baby booties.

6. Give Yourself a Time-Out

Sometimes, mental distraction isn't enough—you need to physically remove yourself from a situation that may simply be too tempting to bear. Just walk away. As in, leave the bar/wedding/funeral/wine-tasting entirely. It'll give you enough time to gather your thoughts, fire up your reserves, and continue to keep the booze at bay. Once you're in a better place, reward yourself. Eat a banana split. Meditate. Work out. Break out the iPod. Take a bath. Have your partner rub cocoa butter on your belly and see where the night takes you.

Apple Pie in a Glass

by Randy Halloran, for the Minnesota Organization on Fetal Alcohol Syndrome's Pregnant Pause Competition

4 oz. frozen apple juice concentrate

1 cup vanilla ice cream

1/4 tsp. ground cinnamon

1 cup milk

1/2 oz. caramel sauce

Blend all ingredients together in a blender. Serve in a clear mug with a spoon and a straw. Recipe makes two servings.

7. Mix up a Magical Mocktail

Now that you've got no shortage of fabulous, firewater-free recipes to choose from, break out the blender and go nuts. It'll satisfy that pesky oral fixation and fill you up fast. Out on the town? Tell that cute bartender you're urgin' for a virgin, and challenge him to serve up his sexiest spiritless specialty.

8. Phone a Friend; Share with Your Shrink

A sympathetic ear is worth its weight in wine. Whether you're the first of your friends to dabble in fertility or not, calling a pal for support is bound to motivate you to do the right thing. Admitting you're feeling momentarily weak will not only make you accountable for your actions to somebody besides yourself, it'll be a source of pride when you successfully kick temptation's ass. If you've got a good therapist, she'll be an able ally, too. She probably knows you better than you know yourself anyway, so let her guide you in the right direction.

9. Buy Something—*Fast!*

Sometimes, replacing one self-destructive act with another is just what the obstetrician ordered. Now's the perfect time to break out that credit card and hit the streets. We're not talking about baby supplies here—you need something just for you. (This applies even when—and especially if—your Visa is already maxed to the hilt with onesies and strollers.) We recommend handbags or makeup or books—you know, the sort of thing that always fits. Feeling too fragile to make it out the door? Log on and max out: there's no shortage of good shopping in cyberspace.

Apricot Punch

From the New Jersey Coalition for Prevention of Developmental Disabilities

Ice

1 oz. cherry juice

2 oz. apricot juice

2 oz. orange juice

2 oz. pineapple juice

Fruit, for garnish

Mix ingredients together in cocktail shaker. Strain into a martini glass and serve, or pour over ice and serve in a rocks glass. Garnish with a cherry, orange slice, or pineapple wedge.

10. Become Obsessed with Clean Living

Since you're obviously the obsessive type, swing that pendulum back in the other direction and hop on. Ditch the Sweet 'n Low for seaweed and your Red Bull for green tea, and pretty soon, alcohol will not only cease to hold any power over you whatsoever, but it may actually inspire a healthy dose of loathing and contempt. Sit around and rub your tummy. Let your gray grow in while you watch the grass grow. Maybe even massage your perineum with grapeseed oil in the hopes of avoiding an episiotomy. All the while, enjoy that feeling of smug superiority over the pesticide-ingesting, non-downward-dogging masses. Don't worry—you can go back to poisoning yourself with all that's good in the world after the kid's born.

11. If You Fall, Get Back on the Wagon Immediately

Experience a minor setback? Don't beat yourself up over it for too long. Get back on that stone-cold-sober horse and ride out the rest of your pregnancy as sober as a judge. Take it one day at a time from now on, and be extra-aware that you're ultra-vulnerable when temptation rears its ugly head. For every situation you master sans margarita, you're one step closer to world domination.

12. Accept Responsibility, Mama

It ain't easy, but nothing worthwhile ever is. Take a deep breath and remember that you're no longer drinking for one, but teetotaling for two. Still not sure? Step over to the mirror and take a good, long look at yourself—you're already a mother. A *good* one, too. And good moms don't drink and gestate.

White Sangria Punch

From the New Jersey Coalition for Prevention of Developmental Disabilities

3 cups club soda

4 cups white grape juice

1 cup pink grapefruit juice

1 tbsp. lime juice

Pink grapefruit slices, for garnish

In a large pitcher, combine grape, grapefruit, and lime juices; refrigerate. Just before serving, add soda water and grapefruit slices. Makes twelve servings.

Wise Words to Inspire the Mother-to-Be

Looking for a little life lesson or just a good laugh to get you through a tough day? The following fine folks said it best, with wit and wisdom to spare…

We gain the strength of the temptation we resist.

—*Ralph Waldo Emerson*

If passion drives you, let reason hold the reins.

—*Ben Franklin*

It's not easy being a mother. If it were easy, fathers would do it.

—*Dorothy Zbornak,* The Golden Girls

Saints are sinners who kept on going.

—*Robert Louis Stevenson*

By far the most common craving of pregnant women is not to be pregnant.

—*Phyllis Diller*

Don't wreck a sublime chocolate experience by feeling guilty. Chocolate isn't like premarital sex. It will not make you pregnant. And it always feels good.

—*Lora Brody*

Birth is not only about making babies. Birth is about making mothers—strong, competent, capable mothers who trust themselves and know their inner strength.

—*Barbara Katz Rothman*

When you are a mother, you are never really alone in your thoughts. A mother always has to think twice, once for herself and once for her child.

—*Sophia Loren*

A mother who is really a mother is never free.

—*Honore de Balzac*

Life is tough enough without having someone kick you from the inside.

—*Rita Rudner*

It has ever been my experience that folks who have no vices have very few virtues. —*Abraham Lincoln*

Do not bite at the bait of pleasure till you know there is no hook beneath it.

—*Thomas Jefferson*

It is good to be without vices, but it is not good to be without temptations.

—*Walter Bage*

A baby's an inestimable blessing and bother.

—*Mark Twain*

When I read about the evils of drinking, I gave up reading.

—*Henry Youngman*

Snappy Comebacks to Stupid Comments

In your battle to stay sober, sane, and safe, you will surely encounter plenty of fools along the road to motherhood. When they open their mouths without thinking, it's tempting to want to rip them a new one. Though it's impossible to remember every single idiotic thing people have said that made us want to throttle them, we've compiled the list below—from the very earliest stages of pregnancy to the awful, overdue end—so you won't be caught off guard when it happens to you.

Here's also what we wish we'd said at the time—sassy ways to let people know they should be minding their own business instead of getting all up in yours. Okay, so maybe they're technically not *all* alcohol-related, but when you're struggling through nine gassy, sleepless, bloated, sober months, any little thing can tick you off, and you need as much ammo as you can get, right?

Just arm yourself with these witty retorts, and you're sure to be prepared the next time somebody comes along with a waistline wisecrack or rude comment about your alcohol consumption. If they take offense, just blame it on your hormones. Do you really care what they think, anyway? (For those times when you might, we've also included a more polite version of the response designed for anyone you really can't afford to offend—no matter how much you may want to!)

Before They Know…
"Your boobs are huge!"

Snarky comeback: "I could say the same thing about your butt!"

Polite reply: "I guess the Wonderbra's working!"

"Did you gain weight?"

Snarky comeback: "No. Your eyes must have shrunk."

Polite reply: "Thanks to all your wonderful cooking!" or "Thanks to that great restaurant you recommended!"

"My lord, are those breast implants?"

Snarky comeback: "Nope—I'm just happy to see you."

Polite reply: "Nope—I'm just lucky to be so well-endowed!"

"You look so tired lately."

Snarky comeback: "I was thinking the same thing about you. Is everything okay?"

Polite reply: "Can you recommend a good cure for insomnia?"

"Your tummy used to be so flat!"

Snarky comeback: "Bloating is a sign of many serious illnesses. Just pick one and spread the word, would you?"

Polite reply: "Thanks. I must have hidden it well, then!"

"You look green. Are you sick?"

Snarky comeback: "Yeah—sick of people telling me I look like crap. Mind your own damn business!"

Polite reply: "I accidentally bought the wrong shade of foundation."

"You look different. Did you do something?"

Snarky comeback: "You mean besides gaining

weight and breaking out?"

Polite reply: "Why, yes—I've been working out. People are really starting to notice!"

"Are you pregnant?"

Snarky comeback: "Well, if I ever do get pregnant, I was planning to tell my husband first, but now that I think about it, you should definitely be the first to know."

Polite reply: "Wouldn't that be nice!" or "Even if I were, I'd be too superstitious to tell anyone before the three-month mark."

At the Bar...

"You're not drinking? Are you trying to get pregnant or something?"

Snarky comeback: "Not drinking alcohol can get you pregnant? Funny—I always thought it was sex…"

Polite reply: "Naw, I'm just saving my calories for the giant piece of chocolate cake waiting for me in my fridge!"

"Why aren't you drinking?"

Snarky comeback: "I'm in a twelve-step program, but thanks for asking."

Polite reply: "I'm worried it'll make my headache worse."

"Let me get you something else—Perrier's not a drink!"

Snarky comeback: "It's not? Do you think they'll give me a refund?"

Polite reply: "I know, but it's still a bit early for me" or "I know, but I already had some wine with lunch."

"You're only having water? Are you on a diet or something?"

Snarky comeback: "Yes. Please tell me which one you're on so I can try another."

Polite reply: "No, I'm just really trying to get in my eight glasses a day."

"You used to be the life of the party! Are you getting boring in your old age?"

Snarky comeback: "I'd rather be boring than rude."

Polite reply: "With age comes wisdom."

"Why'd you order a Shirley Temple?"

Snarky comeback: "Because I'm under twenty-one. How old are you?"

Polite reply: "They're actually quite delicious—let me get you one to try."

At Work...

"You seem tired. Is everything all right?"

Snarky comeback: "Now that you mention it, I'd love to go home early today. Cover for me, okay?"

Polite reply: "I was up late talking to a friend on the West Coast/in Hawaii."

"Have you gained weight?"

Snarky comeback: "It's hard to get to the gym when I work so late every night and come in so early every morning, boss."

Polite reply: "It's that gosh-darn vending machine!"

"What happened to your wardrobe? You used to be so chic!"

Snarky comeback: "I gave all my old clothes to charity, but if I'd known you could have used them, I would have given you first crack."

Polite reply: "I give all my old clothes to charity every few years—it's a great excuse to go shopping for new stuff!"

"You're going home early again?"

Snarky comeback: "You're keeping track? Thanks for caring so much."

Polite reply: "I've been working weekends instead."

Once You're Showing...

"Excuse me, but should you be drinking that if you're pregnant?"

Snarky comeback: "Actually, it's a mocktail—but if you don't mind your own business, the next Bloody Mary around here is gonna be you."

Polite reply: "Wow—this mocktail sure does look like the real thing!"

"Don't be such a party pooper—one drink won't kill the baby!"

Snarky comeback: "Obviously, your mother did it and you turned out fine, right?"

Polite reply: "I like to err on the side of caution when it comes to drinking and pregnancy."

"Come on, have a sip. It's bad luck not to toast with alcohol."

Snarky comeback: "And it's even worse luck to be cursed by a pregnant woman."

Polite reply: "My husband's agreed to have an extra one for me!"

"You're carrying so low/high/large/small!"

Snarky comeback: "Thanks, I think. Now let's talk about your body for a change…"

Polite reply: "It's amazing how the human body changes to accommodate a growing baby!"

"You're so big, you must be carrying twins!"

Snarky comeback: "How did you get so much smarter than the sonogram machine?" or "Actually, I'm carrying small—it's triplets."

Polite reply: "This singleton may look like twins, but it feels more like triplets!"

"Do you know what it is yet?"

Snarky comeback: "Hopefully a baby."

Polite reply: "Don't you just love secrets?"

"Do you want a boy or a girl?"

Snarky comeback: "We're shooting for one or the other."

Polite reply: "We're still just delighted to be expecting."

"You're too old/young to be pregnant!"

Snarky comeback: "You're right. I've got a pillow under my shirt."

Polite reply: "I guess Mother Nature knows best."

"Didn't you just have a baby?"

Snarky comeback: "That would explain the crib in our spare bedroom."

Polite reply: "Yes, and won't it be wonderful for him/her to have a sibling so close in age?"

"Boy, you sure are fertile!"

Snarky comeback: "Boy, you sure are barren."

Polite reply: "We really are blessed to be able to conceive."

"Can you afford a baby?"

Snarky comeback: "Sure—we're going to sell it on eBay to pay the hospital bill."

Polite reply: "Can we afford not to? Children are such a treasure."

PROFESSIONAL HELP:

Where to Turn When You Really Can't Go It Alone

"My hands are shaking, my heart's racing...why am I finding this so hard?"
—*Ilana K., 31, New York, NY*

Let's be honest. No matter how high the stakes are or how awesome your willpower might be, sticking to sobriety is harder for some than for others.

These days, most women have lived a little before finding that perfect partner for procreating. Indeed, many of us accumulated some serious baggage along the way, and we don't mean Louis Vuitton. Now's not the time to let those suitcases weigh heavily on your heart—there's no shortage of amazing moms out there who are already good friends with Bill W. (If you don't know who that is, consider yourself lucky.) But no matter how many weeks, months, years, or even decades of sobriety you may have under your belt, your own impending motherhood will test your dedication to the max.

Pregnancy is bound to be a time of great introspection. Maybe newfound concern for the welfare of that unborn babe has just now made you realize you might have a real drinking problem, or maybe the stress of it all is leading you back down some uglier paths traveled in the past. Thinking about starting your own family can easily reopen childhood wounds and create new strain within your personal and professional relationships. When the most effective stress reliever you've ever known is suddenly off-limits, alcohol becomes more tempting than ever. After all, this is the time when that normally recreational pint of ale would otherwise morph into something medically necessary to prevent a nervous breakdown.

The good news? Realizing you need a little extra support now and taking the necessary steps to get it is what's going to make you an even better mom than you ever thought you could be. Fortunately, there's an embarrassment of riches out there when it comes to help keeping the bottle at bay.

If you just can't go it alone, here are our picks for the best resources out there.

MDs and Midwives

Your first line of defense is your doctor or midwife. In order for him or her to help get you and your baby through your pregnancy happily and healthily, you need to speak honestly and frankly. Sounds scary, we know. But there's nothing to be ashamed of unless you *don't* do what you have to in order to stay clean and sober, for your sake and for that little bun in your oven.

If you're a heavy drinker, the first hurdle might be withdrawal. It's a difficult enough process for those who aren't pregnant, which is why we cannot overstate the importance of talking to a doctor before you begin any recovery program; resolving the physical aspects of alcohol dependency can be especially sensitive during pregnancy for a variety or reasons, and should never be attempted alone.

Not only will your health care professional guide you both safely through the biggest hangover of your life, but he or she will also be able to refer you to a recommended psychologist, addiction specialist, support group, or social worker in your area for the long haul.

Only one recipe in this chapter, inspired by that old sobriety standby—coffee. Make it decaf if you prefer, as long as you keep on trucking.

Sweet and Sober

We named this drink in honor of the reality check you might currently be giving yourself. While we know that coffee has a historical, albeit unfounded, reputation as a way to sober up, it's also a familiar fuel at recovery meetings. The simple truth is, for many of us, the only real way to sober up is to ask for a helping hand. And so, we also added a sweet component to this symbolic drink, to remind you not to be too hard on yourself these days—your commitment to complete sobriety is tough enough. Congratulations on doing the right thing, for you and baby.

6 tbsp. ground coffee, decaf if you prefer

½ cup caramel dessert sauce

4 ½ cups cold water

Prepared whipped topping, thawed, for garnish

2 tbsp. chocolate-covered toffee (aka Skor bar), chopped, for garnish

For those with an automatic coffeemaker, first place caramel sauce in the empty pot of the coffeemaker and prepare coffee as usual (using cold water). When brewing is complete, stir until well-mixed. Makes six servings. For those with coffeemakers that make individual cups, pour about 1 oz. of caramel sauce into coffee mug, brew as usual, and stir. Top each serving with thawed whipped topping and sprinkle with chopped chocolate-covered toffee, if desired.

Support Groups and Recovery Programs
Alcoholics Anonymous

Alcoholics Anonymous is the largest recovery program and self-help group in the world. By many accounts, it is also the most successful. Through a time-tested plan of following the Twelve Steps, one-to-one sponsorship support, and those ubiquitous group meetings, people from every corner of the earth who've struggled with alcohol have found sobriety and compassion in AA for more than seventy years.

Its mandate is simple:

Alcoholics Anonymous is a fellowship of men and women who share their experience, strength, and hope with each other that they may solve their common problem and help others to recover from alcoholism.

The only requirement for membership is a desire to stop drinking. There are no dues or fees for AA membership; we are self-supporting through our own contributions. AA is not allied with any sect, denomination, politics, organization, or institution; does not wish to engage in any controversy; neither endorses nor opposes any causes. Our primary purpose is to stay sober and help other alcoholics to achieve sobriety.

(Copyright © by the AA Grapevine, Inc.; The AA Preamble is reprinted with permission of the AA Grapevine, Inc.)

Though AA is not specifically geared toward pregnant women, its philosophies and programs can easily be adapted to suit the swollen-bellied set. Of the estimated two million people around the world who are currently members of AA, about 35 percent are women, a great many of whom are mothers who've been exactly where you are right now. Some might not have made it through their pregnancies alcohol-free, while others found a way. Either way, their experience will likely be invaluable, whether you're looking for an occasional pat on the shoulder or friendly smile as you work the program, or a full-blown sponsor with whom to build a relationship.

Contact

Alcoholics Anonymous
General Service Office, United States
P.O. Box 459
Grand Central Station
New York, NY 10163
website: www.aa.org
phone: (212) 870–3400

For local links to regional offices, visit the AA website to access online lists of meeting times and phone numbers offering recorded information, or check the white pages of your local phone book under "Alcoholics Anonymous."

Secular Organizations for Sobriety

The not-for-profit Secular Organizations for Sobriety, also known as SOS or Save Our Selves, is one of the most popular alternatives to Alcoholics Anonymous. Though equally anonymous and also focusing on peer-based support and meetings, SOS emphasizes the importance of rational decision-making, self-reliance, and the desire to keep religion and spirituality out of recovery, and therefore offers an effective alternative for those who are uncomfortable with the "Higher Power" aspect of most twelve-step programs.

Contact
Secular Organizations for Sobriety
4773 Hollywood Boulevard
Hollywood, CA 90027
website: www.sossobriety.org or www.cfiwest.org/sos
phone:(323) 666–4295

Smart Recovery

SMART Recovery, aka Self-Management and Recovery Training, also offers a religion-free alternative to achieving sobriety, with an emphasis on proven cognitive behavioral therapy techniques. The SMART Four-Point Program employs scientific and evidence-based methods (sort of a brains-over-beer kind of approach), and is constantly evolving to incorporate new research in the field of alcohol and addiction recovery. Hundreds of face-to-face meetings and frequent online SMART groups provide support.

Contact

SMART Recovery

7537 Mentor Avenue, Suite 306

Mentor, OH 44060

website: www.smartrecovery.org

phone: (440) 951–5357

toll-free: 1–866–951–5357

Women for Sobriety

According to Women for Sobriety (WFS)—the first women-only self-help group for overcoming problem drinking—there are seven and a half million female alcoholics living in the United States today. The non-profit organization was formed to address the particular emotional and psychological needs of women in recovery, so their members boast a wealth of experience when it comes to drinking and pregnancy. The WFS "New Life Acceptance" program, based on thirteen affirmations, promotes positive reinforcement and thinking, as well as physical support via diet, exercise, meditation, and relaxation. The hundreds of local WFS support groups also place a high priority on anonymity, as does the thriving online WFS community at msn.com.

Contact

Women for Sobriety
P.O. Box 618
Quakertown, PA 18951–0618
website: www.womenforsobriety.org
MSN group: http://groups.msn.com/WomenforSobriety
phone: (215) 536–8026

Rational Recovery

Rational Recovery offers an entirely different approach to sobriety in that it promotes "self-recovery." It vehemently opposes twelve-step programs, group meetings, and religion within the recovery setting, and sees alcoholism as a bad habit, not a disease. Proponents of RR say that instead of depending on other people or a higher power for support, the best way to beat alcohol addiction is to find strength from within. RR's free, self-directed program of abstinence and self-control—known as AVRT, or Addictive Voice Recognition Technique—is available on its website.

Contact

Rational Recovery
Box 800
Lotus, CA 95651
website: www.rational.org
phone: (530) 621–2667 or (530) 621–4374

Counseling and Treatment Referral Services
National Council on Alcoholism and Drug Dependence

The National Council on Alcoholism and Drug Dependence (NCADD) is a privately funded organization that has been fighting the stigma of alcoholism by educating the public, advising the government, and offering information and support for more than sixty years to those with drinking problems. Through its website, it maintains an extensive list of local affiliates that provide referrals to addiction counselors and group-treatment facilities. The service is also accessible twenty-four hours a day via its toll-free Hope Line.

Contact

National Council on Alcoholism and Drug Dependence
22 Cortlandt Street, Suite 801
New York, NY 10007–3128
website: www.ncadd.org
phone: (212) 269–7797
Hope Line: 1–800-NCA-CALL

Substance Abuse and Mental Health Services Administration

SAMHSA—the Substance Abuse and Mental Health Services Administration, a branch of the U.S. Department of Health and Human Services—is a tremendous source of information on virtually all addiction and mental-health problems. Broadly stated, the agency's main goal is to improve the lives of people suffering from these afflictions, and to that end, it offers an excellent search engine on its website (also accessible by phone through its Referral Helpline) listing approved drug- and alcohol-abuse treatment centers in your neighborhood, whether you hail from Georgia or Guam.

Contact

Substance Abuse and Mental Health Services
  Administration
1 Choke Cherry Road
Rockville, MD 20850
main website: www.samhsa.gov
Substance Abuse Treatment Facility Locator:
  http://findtreatment.samhsa.gov
Referral Helpline: 1–800–662-HELP

The American Council on Alcoholism

The American Council on Alcoholism (ACA) is a national nonprofit outreach and educational organization—basically, one-stop shopping for anyone with a drinking problem who wants to get sober. Information on alcohol, the latest research into various treatments, and an online self-screening test make the ACA website tops. Toll-free, twenty-four-hour access to a help- and treatment-referral line allows callers to find effective, affordable help fast. Taking that difficult first step doesn't get any easier than this.

Contact

American Council on Alcoholism
1000 E. Indian School Road
Phoenix, AZ 85014
website: www.acausa.org
Helpline: 1–800–527–5344

Substance Safety

Motherisk

Motherisk is a public-health initiative run by Toronto's Hospital for Sick Children, and is uniquely dedicated to providing pregnant women, employers, and medical professionals with an authoritative source for exactly what is and is not safe to be exposed to during pregnancy, from house paint and herbs to illnesses and industrial by-products. Its expertise is backed by the latest research, with new studies constantly underway, and is available to the public via its various publications, an exhaustive new website, and several helplines. If you can't make it to the on-site Motherisk Clinic, calm and reassuring counseling and answers to questions about alcohol for pregnant and lactating women are available by phone.

Contact

Motherisk Program
Hospital for Sick Children
555 University Avenue
Toronto, ON M5G 1X8
website: www.motherisk.org
phone: (416) 813–6780

National Toxicology Program

The National Toxicology Program (NTP), run by the National Institute of Environmental Health Sciences (NIEHS), is dedicated to protecting the safety of the public by evaluating risks posed by various chemical and substances to human health. Its **Center for the Evaluation of Risks to Human Reproduction (CERHR)** is entrusted with all fertility, gestational, and developmental issues, and is a valuable voice on the safety of exposure to various substances during pregnancy. The CERHR also has a section on its website devoted to the risks of alcohol during pregnancy.

Contact

Center for the Evaluation of Risks to Human
  Reproduction
NIEHS EC-32
P.O. Box 12233
Research Triangle Park, NC 27709

NTP website: http://ntp.niehs.nih.gov
CERHR website: http://cerhr.niehs.nih.gov
CERHR alcohol page:
  http://cerhr.niehs.nih.gov/common/alcohol.html
phone: (919) 541–3455

Pregnant Pause

Pregnant Pause is an initiative of The Arc—a national advocacy coalition of statewide chapters devoted to improving the lives of kids and adults with developmental disabilities, many the result of alcohol-exposed pregnancies. The Pregnant Pause campaign, begun by The Arc, New Jersey, and since adopted by many other state chapters, raises public and media awareness of the hazards of drinking and gestating by organizing fun community events, such as nonalcoholic drink contests at local bars judged by pregnant women (we've included a few of the winners in Chapter 6!) and free baby showers. Your local ARC chapter, which can be found through the national website, will have information on events near you.

Contact

The ARC of the United States
1010 Wayne Avenue, Suite 650
Silver Spring, MD 20910
website: www.thearc.org
phone: (301) 565–3842

Fetal Alcohol Syndrome

National Organization on Fetal Alcohol Syndrome

The National Organization on Fetal Alcohol Syndrome (NOFAS) is the number-one authority on alcohol-related birth defects. It also acts as an advocate for families and expectant mothers dealing with related issues, and runs extensive public- and professional-education programs in the hope of furthering prevention. Its website contains plenty of up-to-date information on the risks associated with drinking and gestating, plus a comprehensive and easily accessible collection of the latest research on the subject.

Contact

National Organization on Fetal Alcohol Syndrome
900 17th Street NW, Suite 910
Washington, DC 20006
website: www.nofas.org
phone: (202) 785–4585
toll-free: 1–800–66–NOFAS

March of Dimes

The world's leading nonprofit organization dedicated to research into and the prevention of birth defects, prematurity, and infant mortality is the March of Dimes. Its website has a ton of advice on how to enjoy a safe and healthy pregnancy, some general information about alcohol and other big no-nos, as well as an in-depth Fact Sheet designed for professionals but which you may find helpful since it's an excellent overview of all the relevant issues.

Contact

March of Dimes
1275 Mamaroneck Avenue
White Plains, NY 10605
website: www.marchofdimes.com
Alcohol and Pregnancy Fact Sheet:
www.marchofdimes.com/professionals/681_1170.asp
phone: (914) 997–4488
toll-free: 1–888–MODIMES

Samhsa's Fetal Alcohol Spectrums Disorder (FASD) Center for Excellence

Aside from its comprehensive Substance Abuse Treatment Facility Locator (discussed on page 187), SAMHSA—the Substance Abuse and Mental Health Services Administration—runs the Fetal Alcohol Spectrums Disorder (FASD) Center for Excellence. The federally funded Center focuses on the specific problems of alcohol-related birth defects and disorders, as well as prevention and education among health care professionals, educators, women of childbearing age, and the general public. The FASD Center has an information line and also offers an exhaustive searchable database of books, websites, and newspaper and journal articles.

Contact

SAMHSA FASD Center for Excellence

2101 Gaither Road, Suite 600

Rockville, MD 20850

website: www.fasdcenter.samhsa.gov

phone: 1–866–STOPFAS

Centers For Disease Control and Prevention

The CDC's National Center on Birth Defects and Developmental Disabilities (NCBDDD) has an excellent webpage on Fetal Alcohol Spectrum Disorders—containing all the latest research, government initiatives, and information for families on the wide range of problems that may result from alcohol-exposed pregnancies, with a focus on prevention and intervention.

Contact

Fetal Alcohol Syndrome

NCBDDD, CDC

Mail-Stop E-86

1600 Clifton Road

Atlanta, GA 30333

website: www.cdc.gov/ncbddd/fas

phone: 1–800–CDC–INFO

The United States Department of Health and Human Services

While most of us believe the government should pretty much steer clear of our bedrooms and admire our burgeoning bellies from afar, several of its agencies—functioning under the vast umbrella of the U. S. Department of Health and Human Services (HHS)—offer a veritable treasure trove of no-nonsense information when it comes to drinking, pregnancy, and alcohol addiction.

Surgeon General's Warning

Wondering where the Surgeon General—the country's leading spokesperson on public health—stands on drinking and pregnancy? Richard H. Carmona, who held the position until recently, released the Department of Health and Human Services's position on the subject on February 1, 2005. The current news release replaces an outdated and vaguely worded 1981 Surgeon General's Advisory that simply recommended that pregnant women limit the amount of alcohol they consume.

Contact

Office of the Surgeon General

5600 Fishers Lane

Room 18–66

Rockville, MD 20857

main website: www.surgeongeneral.gov

Access the new Advisory at www.hhs.gov/surgeon general/pressreleases/sg02222005.html

National Institute on Alcohol Abuse and Alcoholism

The National Institute on Alcohol Abuse and Alcoholism (NIAAA) is that branch of the National Institutes of Health entrusted with researching all things alcoholic and disseminating those findings to the public, government, and educational sectors. It is also committed to finding a way to reduce the incidence of Fetal Alcohol Syndrome on a national level through its **Interagency Coordinating Committee on Fetal Alcohol Syndrome** (ICCFAS), which coordinates the efforts of the many government bodies involved in the fight against FAS in order to improve their efficacy.

Contact

National Institute on Alcohol Abuse and Alcoholism
5635 Fishers Lane
MSC 9304
Bethesda, MD 20892–9304
website: www.niaaa.nih.gov
ICCFAS website:
 www.niaaa.nih.gov/AboutNIAAA/Interagency

Alcohol Policy Information System

The Alcohol Policy Information System (APIS), an initiative of the NIAAA, provides concise and up-to-date details on state and federal laws regarding alcohol. If you're curious what the regulations are in your state regarding pregnant women who drink, for example, or what the reporting requirements are for health professionals, head to the "Policy Topics Index" on the APIS website and click on "Alcohol and Pregnancy" for the answers.

Contact
website: www.alcoholpolicy.niaaa.nih.gov
for further information: info@apis.cdmgroup.com

chapter

8

PARTAKING POSTPARTUM:

Crossing the Finish Line

"I had a beer or two and now my baby seems
drunk! Is it just me?"
—*Robyn B., 25, Boston, MA*

You did it! You made it through nine long, anxiety-wracked months sober, safe, and seriously addicted to spa services and chocolate. Okay, so there were a few rough moments in there, but all that's behind you now—your baby's cradled safely in your arms, healthy as a horse, and you want to keep it that way. On the other hand, you've been *sooo* good for *sooo* long...

So what now?

Here's where the line gets a little fuzzy, and we're not talking about that horrible linea negra snaking down your suddenly deflated belly. Is the prohibition lifted postpartum, or is alcohol still entirely off-limits for the foreseeable future? Only you can decide for sure. The answers to the following queries about consuming during your confinement (and beyond) will help you do just that, you responsible new mother, you.

Even though you no longer have baby on board, you certainly won't be partaking alone. We've included several recipes here—inspired by whatever season junior was born in—to serve to larger groups, since chances are your house will be flooded with friends and family anxious to meet the new addition. (Nonalcoholic punches will also allow breast-feeders and big brothers and sisters to participate in all the toasting.) And last but certainly not least, our final recipe is the perfect way to rekindle your romance with your real significant other—alcohol.

Winter Baby

Try this recipe to toast your winter baby's December arrival, or if you're actually up for hosting that holiday party at your place. It's evidence that even without the raw eggs and alcohol—both of which are off-limits—it can still taste like eggnog!

8 cups milk

1 (3 oz.) package of French-vanilla instant pudding

up to ½ cup sugar

2 tsp. vanilla extract

½ tsp. nutmeg

In a large bowl, mix the pudding with 1 cup of the milk. When pudding is formed, add in the remaining ingredients (slowly adding sugar and tasting as you go) and mix very well. Chill and serve.

Time for a Taste

Q: *"How soon is too soon to resume? As in, can I have a drink before the epidural wears off?"*

Ah, a complicated question, grasshopper.

Most hospitals will officially frown on that bottle of Dom that Daddy wants to pop in the delivery room. But, as with any rule worth breaking, the risks may be worth the reward. Once you're all cleaned up, the legion of medical personnel who attended the birth will likely leave you alone to bond, breast-feed, and/or secretly break open the bubbly. This is also when impatient grandparents, friends, and relatives will storm the room, anxious to meet the new addition and toast his or her arrival.

As for you, you'll probably be wasted already. Any combination of epidural anesthesia, cervical blocks, nitrous oxide, opioids, pethidine, sleep deprivation, and adrenaline makes for a pretty intoxicating experience, and it's unlikely you'll be up for any major partying at this point. But if it's going around, by all means have a sip, if just to symbolize the end of one era and to celebrate the beginning of a new one. Having more than that is not a great idea, since any drug strong enough to make childbirth pleasant is obviously contraindicated to alcohol consumption.

What's that? You did it...*naturally?* No painkillers at all? Seriously? Well, then—our hats are off to you. By all means, have an entire *bottle* of champagne. You can even send us the bill.

Q: *"After all this time, will my tolerance have changed?"*

Probably. Or at least your interpretation of it will have, so attuned (and appreciative) will you be of even the slightest alcoholic buzz. Of course, all sorts of factors can come into play here as well, such as your exhaustion level, how much weight you're hanging onto, and how desperate you are to feel no pain. In general, though, a state of tipsiness previously attainable in two drinks may suddenly be achieved in one. Our recommendation? After forty long weeks without, enjoy the fact that you're now a cheap date and break out the good cognac.

Q: *"Now that we're home from the hospital, can I finally resume happy hour?"*

Guess what? Happy hour is now any consecutive sixty-minute period in which you are asleep. What you think you are referring to will, from this point forward, be known as Mommy Time. That elusive beast goes by many other names as well, such as Shower, Baby-sitter, and Lunch.

If you're bottle-feeding, the good news is that once you're home from the hospital and have weaned yourself off any postpartum painkillers, the bar is finally open. Try not to be too shocked when you realize the hard part's really just beginning; now that baby's ex-utero, it's actually *tougher* to keep him or her safe in the real world. As you settle into your new life together, remember to always drink responsibly. The last thing junior needs is a mother who can't find the tip of her nose with her left hand and slurs her ga-ga goo-goos.

If you're breast-feeding, then an entirely different set of rules comes into play. So for all you lactating lovelies out there, the following section will cover everything you need to know about alcohol and nursing.

Breast-feeding Issues: Tipple and the Nipple

By now, we're sure you've heard it a hundred times: nursing your little one is a great idea. Not only is your milk the perfect food for baby, but it also offers some other benefits that can't be beat. There's the bonding, of course, not to mention the sheer convenience of it (no bottles or formula to contend with), the drop-the-baby-weight factor (nursing exclusively burns up to five hundred calories a day!), and the delay of the return of your period (major plus). Some studies also suggest benefits to your bones, as well as reduced rates of both ovarian cancer and premenopausal breast cancer.

While breast-feeding may very well be one of the best things you can do for both you and baby, it can also be a challenge. For example, contrary to what you may have heard, nursing does *not* come naturally to every new mother; indeed, for many of us it is more of a learned art than an instinct. Before getting the hang of it for good, lots of newly nursing moms will contend with cracked nipples, engorgement, bad latches, supply problems (too much milk or too little milk), those blasted breast pumps, tied tongues, hideous bras, plugged ducts, mastitis, thrush...alas, the list goes on and on. So why do we do it? Simple: the pains are often worth the gains.

Still, the last thing a new mom weighing the pros and cons needs is another check in the "Reasons Not To" column, which is why we're switching "Drinking" back to the plus side. Many people mistakenly believe that nursing mothers need to maintain that mentally exhausting gestational hypervigilance on what goes into or onto their bodies until baby's been weaned. With a few notable exceptions, like certain drugs, this simply isn't true. Although lots of what you eat does leach into your milk supply (that's the idea, right?), there's simply no evidence to suggest that the *responsible* consumption of alcohol is in any way detrimental to the mental, emotional, or physical health of your baby.

Phew!

So, what exactly do we mean by responsible? Read on for the answers.

Q: *"If I drink, will there be enough alcohol in my milk to harm my baby in any way?"*

That depends—did you drink a case of twelve beers every day for a month, or did you have half a raspberry wine cooler with lunch last Tuesday? In other words, how much you drink and how often you drink it is what will determine the effect that alcohol will have on your kid. Your weight, body fat, food intake, and general tolerance level also help determine your blood-alcohol level, and therefore how much booze reaches your milk. In general, the alcohol level in your milk is roughly equivalent to the alcohol level in your blood at any given time.

Because of this, even if you breast-feed at that moment when the alcohol level in your milk peaks, your baby isn't really being exposed to that much alcohol at all. The second-hand effects of that magical, minty mojito on the baby are temporary and primarily sedative, including possible drowsiness and poorer sucking, as well as a reduction in your milk-ejection (or let-down) reflex and decreased milk production.

The consequences of a nursing mother's alcohol intake become more of a problem when she drinks frequently over time, since a sleepy, weakly sucking baby with access to poorly functioning breasts eats not only less often, but takes in less milk at each meal. As the weeks pass, this can cause a failure to thrive, poor weight gain, general weakness, hypoglycemia, and impairments in neuro-motor development, all of which have been noted in the babies of moms who are moderate to heavy drinkers. There is also some evidence to suggest that alcohol might change the way milk smells and tastes, something which, over time, may also lower baby's milk intake and tinker with mom's production.

The age of your little one is another factor to consider. Babies under three months old have immature livers, which means that any alcohol they're exposed to—even the limited amounts passed on via breast milk—stays in their systems longer and may have a greater effect on them. Because of this, some moms decide to wait till their babies are no longer infants before they resume drinking.

Sounds scary, we know.

But provided you're not boozing it up all day long, there's really no reason to be overly concerned (most sources seem to agree on an upward limit of one drink per day, *occasionally* two). Both the American Academy of Pediatrics and La Leche League (the world's largest breast-feeding support network, information source, and advocacy group)—neither of which are in the business of putting babies at risk—state that the occasional drink is just fine for nursing moms, especially if they keep their breasts to themselves for roughly two to three hours after partaking.

The safest way to drink and lactate responsibly is to let your liver do its thing and wait for the alcohol in your blood (and therefore your milk) to be disposed of before feeding the baby. Coffee, drinking lots of water, and/or pumping and dumping won't help you or your milk sober up any quicker, by the way—that's just an old drunk wives' tale. Time is the only thing that filters out whatever fun you've been having.

Q: *"So, you're saying my baby actually can get drunk off my milk if I don't wait to sober up?"*

Yup! Although the amount of alcohol in your breast milk is relatively low, when your tiny four-week-old and her immature liver knock back a few ounces of your martini-laced milk, you may notice she's suddenly unable to walk a straight line. Kidding!…sort of. As we pointed out a little earlier, alcohol does have a sedative effect on the breast-fed baby. She may seem sleepy, generally drowsy, unable to suck well, or uninterested in nursing.

We know, we know—the prospect of a sleepy baby sounds almost as good as that Tequila Sunrise tastes. Despite your understandable desire to drug your child into submission, you should probably plan ahead if you intend to drink, and pump a bottle to give to her in case she gets hungry before the booze has left your system. If you're not doing the bottle thing, or you have no extra milk on hand, don't worry too much—aside from a slight hangover, your little devil should be just fine.

And remember: whether you're just a teensy bit tipsy or three sheets to the wind, please refrain from walking around with the baby while intoxicated. A fall is definitely far more dangerous than a little tipple from the nipple any day.

Q: *"Okay, so exactly how long does alcohol stay in my breast milk?"*

Basically, as soon as the effects *you* felt from that vodka gimlet are gone, it's okay to whip out the boob— say two to three hours after you've had one drink (double that for every glass you consume). No need to worry that it stays there until you either pump it or the baby eats, either—like the alcohol in your blood, the alcohol in your milk is metabolized and therefore eliminated over time.

Naturally, other circumstances are relevant, too. If you're imbibing on a full stomach, the alcohol level in your milk reaches its apex from an hour to an hour and half after that drink; if you're running on empty, it's about half that. You can maximize your downtime by giving your kid a bottle of previously stored breast milk, or feeding the baby while you drink (or right after). This will give your body the longest possible window to sober up before it's time to breast-feed again. If you're uncomfortable or overly engorged in the meantime, you could always pump or express a little milk and discard it.

Spring Baby

These days, it seems like everything's growing—except you, for a change! Yes, now that your little lamb is here, you need something bubbly and fruity and fun to celebrate the season. This sparkly concoction makes a delightful stand-in for more spirited punches, and is perfect for a welcome-the-baby party.

3 (3-oz.) packages cherry gelatin

9 cups boiling water

4 cups sugar

4 cups water

2 (46-oz.) cans pineapple juice

6 oz. frozen orange juice concentrate, thawed

4 tbsp. lemon juice

1 (2-liter) bottle ginger ale

In a large pot or saucepan, dissolve the gelatin. In a pot, create a simple syrup by boiling together the sugar and water until the sugar dissolves. In a separate bowl, mix the pineapple juice, orange juice concentrate, and lemon juice. Once the simple syrup is cool, slowly add to the juice mixture (tasting as you go to avoid over-sweetening). Cool. Combine the gelatin and juice mixtures. Pour into plastic containers and freeze (you can prepare this well in advance of the event). Set out to thaw about four to five hours before serving, then add the ginger ale just before serving (the punch will be slushy). Makes twenty-six cups.

Q: *"How many drinks can my baby safely tolerate if I time it just right?"*

Who really knows? The ethical problems of doing studies on drunk moms and their tipsy offspring are too numerous to mention, so exact answers to questions like this can't really be known. Don't take any chances. Your liver probably couldn't process any more than two drinks before it would be time for the kid to eat again, unless you were feeding her from a bottle, so let's leave it at that.

Need to be scared straight? Okay, you asked for it— both binge-drinking and alcoholism in lactating women have been shown to cause problems in their babies. In one case, a single bottle of wine consumed over a twenty-four-hour period caused a baby to sleep constantly, be unable to suck, and feel no pain. Aside from problems with weight gain and neuro-motor development, some breast-fed babies of alcoholics have also been known to exhibit Pseudo-Cushing's Syndrome—involving short stature, moon face, and obesity—though the effects seem to be reversed when the exposure to alcohol ceases.

Since the precise effects of substantial and/or prolonged alcohol exposure via breast milk on the baby's growing brain have not been well-established, a safe threshold cannot be definitively determined. This is clearly not the time to be playing fast and loose with your kid's development; if you find the frequency of your drinking creeping up again now that the baby's been born, seek out some additional help. Talk to your doctor or midwife for a referral to someone who can help, or turn back to Chapter 6, "Sobriety Support," for plenty of tips for getting a handle on problem drinking, as well as a comprehensive list of related resources.

Q: *"Will drinking alcohol help boost my milk supply?"*

Lactation consultants and mothers-in-law have long been telling nursing moms that a little beer or a glass of wine will help your body produce *more* milk. Though we'd love to believe it, this simply isn't the case. What alcohol *does* do is adversely affect a nursing woman's hormone levels, leading to a negative impact on lactation.

In terms of sheer volume, as few as one or two alcoholic drinks seem to have an immediate effect on reducing daily supply, in some cases by nearly a quarter. The research suggests that alcohol causes a significant increase in prolactin, one of the hormones responsible for milk production. More prolactin may mean it takes longer for the body to create milk, as well as cause the *sensation* that one's breasts are full—probably what's responsible for alcohol's ill-founded rep for upping production.

As for its impact on the milk-ejection or let-down reflex, alcohol reduces levels of oxytocin, that feel-good hormone that gets your milk flowing. Because of this, alcohol seems to increase the amount of time it takes from when baby starts sucking to when milk is actually released from the nipple, as well as generally reduce the amount of milk produced.

The sum result of alcohol on your milk? Baby drinks less overall and mom's body produces less—a cycle that can lead to an inadequate supply. Again, this would only become a problem with moderate to heavy alcohol intake, say if you're drinking before every feeding—a tempting thought for those moms experiencing latch-on difficulties or nipple pain!—though the occasional glass of wine here or there is highly unlikely to negatively affect your supply and/or let-down in the medium or long term.

Summer Baby

It's hot and sweaty and you need a drink. Even if you're not having a ton of people over, whip up a batch of sweet, citrusy cooler for yourself and get drunk on vitamin C.

Ice

8 cups cold water

2 cans (12-oz. each) frozen orange juice concentrate, thawed

2 cans (12-oz. each) frozen grapefruit juice concentrate, thawed

2 liters sparkling water, chilled

Mix all ingredients in a large punch bowl. Serve over ice.

Makes thirty servings.

Q: *"So I shouldn't wean my baby because I want to drink more?"*

Not unless you're interested in encouraging the "Trotter Hypothesis." You see, about two hundred years ago, a British doctor named Thomas Trotter conducted a study to see if babies who were weaned off the boob really early on tended to become alcoholics later in life. He found that less breast-feeding did indeed lead to significantly higher rates of problem drinking in adulthood. Several more recent long-term studies seem to back this up, even when accounting for many of the other influential environmental variables that may lead to alcoholism. So, in one of life's delicious little ironies, your breasts, boozy milk and all, may actually help make your baby more immune from a battle with the bottle later on. Trust us—she'll thank you in thirty years when she's pregnant and totally not needing this book.

Ah, the circle of life.

Seriously, though, there's no need to let alcohol get in the way of a successful breast-feeding relationship between you and your baby, because the benefits of nursing definitely outweigh the risks of the responsible enjoyment of cocktails. Unnecessarily restrictive lifestyles and unrealistic fears shouldn't discourage you from breast-feeding, provided, of course, that's what you want to do.

Safety, Alcohol, and Infant Security

Before you got pregnant, the only person you had to worry about when you were drinking was you, assuming you left the car keys alone and the off-key drinking songs to a minimum. Alcohol is a controlled substance, not only because it can be dangerous to the imbiber in large enough quantities, but because the impaired judgment and coordination that result from one too many can be hazardous to those around you. Accepting this basic truth is a responsibility we higher-functioning members of society take very seriously: it's why we don't drink and drive, drink and operate heavy machinery, drink and operate on other people, drink and dial, drink and ski, drink and…well, you get the idea.

It's also why we don't drink and parent, for the most part. In the early weeks or months, when sleep deprivation and recovery from the delivery present real physical obstacles, you may feel that continuing to eschew alcohol is the wisest choice for you and your new family. If you do decide to abstain during the so-called fourth trimester, just stick to the same guidelines and suggestions we've been preaching since page one. With a clean environment and supportive family and friends around you, you can keep on trucking sans sambuca for as long as you need to.

No?

You're ready to start right away?

Okay, okay. We've got you covered.

The good news, of course, is now that baby's out here in the real world, you *can* take a night off from all that responsible teetotaling once in a while. As your kid gets a bit older and you get a bit wiser, life may one day come close to resuming some semblance of normalcy. That means Mommy gets to unwind once again, enjoy a drink with dinner, maybe, or even drown her sorrows for the hell of it from time to time.

When you do finally decide to throw yourself off the wagon, please ensure that the following six extremely important conditions are met:

1. Your tolerance may be much lower, so be vigilant: Tipsy is fun, but totally wasted is not going to end pretty.

2. You're not alone: Make sure Daddy's there to keep an eye on things and help put everyone to bed. Also, since drunk mothers have been known to sleep through the loudest of cries, an extra set of ears is an absolute must.

3. Your significant other is committed to staying relatively sober: At least, sober enough to properly take care of anybody who happens to need a diaper change or who wakes up screaming all of a sudden for no apparent reason (again, this might be either you or the child).

4. You don't get so drunk that it impairs your ability to function for the foreseeable future: The hangover from hell, three middle-of-the-night feedings, and the grossest diaper you've ever encountered make for a Morning After of nuclear proportions.

5. You make the necessary arrangements for breast-fed babies: Either have a bottle of pumped milk on hand, or plan your drinks around feedings so that there's time for the alcohol to clear your system.

6. You use protection: Not to be blunt, but are you really ready to go cold turkey for another nine months so soon?

Fall Baby

Nothing symbolizes fertility like the apple, and this punch incorporates the best flavors of autumn in a party-friendly format. If you like, add a little cinnamon to spice things up.

1 (32-oz.) bottle apple juice, chilled

1 (12-oz.) can frozen cranberry juice concentrate, thawed

1 cup orange juice

1 ½ liters ginger ale

1 apple

In a large punch bowl, combine apple juice, cranberry juice concentrate, and orange juice. Stir until the concentrate has dissolved, then slowly pour in the ginger ale. Thinly slice the apple vertically, forming whole slices. Float apple slices on top of punch. Makes twelve servings.

The Finish Line

No matter when you decide to have that first drink at long last, we believe it's a momentous occasion, and one worth celebrating with pomp and circumstance. If you're lucky enough to snag a baby-sitter this early on in the game, we recommend you hit a nice French restaurant. A big glass of red wine seems somehow a very elegant way to rekindle your romance with the bottle, *oui?* Or, you could head back to your favorite club and dance the night away. Here, there, anywhere…immersing yourself in the outside world will feel great. It'll recharge your batteries, help you reconnect with your significant other, and give you some much-needed time away from you-know-who, even though you'll probably spend most of the night talking about the consistency of your little angel's poop and saying things like "Can you believe *we* have a *kid?*"

More likely, though, you're stuck at home amid a mountain range of rancid laundry and plastic-wrapped dirty-diaper sausages courtesy of that odious, odorous disposal unit. Don't let the indignity of your surroundings spoil the moment: you've been waiting a long time for this drink—*the* drink—so no matter how bleak your current circumstances, it certainly calls for something a little special, doesn't it?

Make sure the baby's asleep, change out of your sweats, light a few candles, put on some soft music. Tonight, let romance reign once again! No matter if it leads to the bedroom or not—and let's face it, it likely won't—you'll just be glad for the chance to slow down and simply appreciate the moment as you savor that first taste of heaven, whether it be an ice-cold beer or a cocktail of epic proportions. Toast each other, your new little love, and your new life together.

For the past nine months, your complete and utter devotion to your unborn child has been nothing short of inspirational. In honor of your smashing success in quelling your compulsion to quaff, we have created a very special, extra-quenching, *real* drink recipe, just for you. And while it may not entirely slake a thirst forty weeks in the making, we feel it's a damn fine start.

So, here's to you, Mom—may you and your new family enjoy all the bountiful blessings a baby brings into the home, and many more years of raising your glasses in good times to come.

The Baby-Bottle Cosmo

Baby bottles can be a convenient way to feed your little bundle of joy, and their handy by-the-ounce gradations mean they make for some pretty nifty cocktail shakers, too. This redefinition of the classic Cosmopolitan is the perfect way to ease back onto the bar stool now that you're ready. Of course, using the bottle to mix it is half the fun. Just make sure you give the symbolic goblet a good washing before passing it back to baby.

2 oz. vodka—at last!

1 oz. Triple Sec

1 oz. cranberry juice

$\frac{1}{2}$ oz. lime juice, fresh squeezed

Pour ingredients into baby bottle. Add ice, shake, and either pour into a rocks glass or strain into a martini glass. If you can't wait, drink it straight out of the bottle!

MOCKTAILS ON THE GO

Don't mourn a restaurant outing for lack of something good to drink—just take your favorite recipes with you! Let's assume that most bartenders (even the knuckleheads) will know how to make the virgin classics—the Bloody Shames, the virgin coladas, and the juice and soda drinks. It's the others that can get a little more complicated. To help you (and them) out, we've jotted down a few copies of these concoctions to carry along on your excursions. We picked drinks to cover a variety of occasions, and those with ingredients most bars are likely to stock. Alternatively, write down your own favorites and bring those with you as well. You may also want to call ahead to see if they have all the necessary ingredients in-house; it might be the first time someone BYO'ed white grape juice for a mock champagne (well worth it!), but who cares? You're pregnant!

Bugs Bunny Special

Ice

3 oz. carrot juice

3 oz. apple juice

Mix portions together in equal parts and serve in a highball glass, on ice.

Absolutely Not

Ice

1 ½ oz. tonic water

6 oz. (ish) orange juice

Cherries, for garnish

First, fill highball glass with ice. Pour in tonic and then fill glass to the top with orange juice.

Spring Mint

Ice   6 sprigs fresh mint

2 oz. Rose's Lime Juice   club soda, to fill

2 oz. simple syrup   Lime wedges, for garnish

Take a martini shaker and add mint, lime juice, and syrup. Fill shaker halfway with ice. Cap and shake so that the mint is broken into little pieces, pour into a collins glass, then fill the rest with soda. Garnish with lime.

Cranberry Cooler

Ice

3 oz. sweet and sour mix

3 oz. cranberry juice

Pineapple wedge, for garnish

Fill a wine glass with ice and pour in the sweet and sour mix and the cranberry juice. Garnish with a pineapple wedge.

Nursery Fizz

Ice

3 oz. ginger ale

3 oz. orange juice

1 splash simple syrup, or a pinch of powdered sugar

cherries and orange slices, for garnish

Fill a large wine glass with ice and pour in all the ingredients. Garnish with a cherry and an orange slice.

Virgin Mai Tai

Ice

4 oz. pineapple juice

2 oz. orange juice

2 oz. club soda

1 tablespoon cream of coconut

1 tablespoon grenadine

Cherries, for garnish

Pour ingredients into a cocktail shaker and shake. Pour into a collins glass, adding additional ice if necessary, and garnish with a cherry and an umbrella.

Sweet Tart

Ice

2 oz. cranberry juice

2 oz. ginger ale

2 oz. lemonade

Mix ingredients in a cocktail shaker with ice and strain into a shooter glass. Ask patron if she prefers it in a wine glass or as a shooter.

Off-White Russian

Ice

$3/4$ oz. simple syrup

$3/4$ oz. cold coffee

4 oz. whole milk

Fill a rocks glass with ice. First mix simple syrup and coffee; then add milk. Ask patron if she prefers to add a scoop of ice cream, if you have it.

Sexless in the City
(aka Virgin Manhattan)

Ice	I tsp. maraschino cherry juice
2 oz cranberry juice	$1/4$ tsp. lemon juice
2 oz orange juice	I–2 dashes orange bitters

Add ingredients to your cocktail shaker and shake. Serve on the rocks in an old-fashioned glass. Garnish with a couple of maraschino cherries.

INDEX

About the Authors

Jackie Rose

Jackie is the author of two internationally acclaimed novels, *Slim Chance* and *Marrying Up*. She continues to put her English lit degree from McGill University to good use in her capacity as a celebrity fashion analyst for *Us Weekly* magazine. Quite amazingly, her broad experience with alcohol has resulted in only a single aversion—Southern Comfort. Jackie lives in Montreal with her husband, Dan, their four-year-old daughter, Abigail, and one-year-old son, Asher.

Caroline Angel, RN, PhD

Caroline Angel, RN, PhD, is a certified mixologist and cosmopolitan aficionado. She holds a doctorate of philosophy in Nursing and Criminology from the University of

Pennsylvania (where she now teaches) and lives in Westfield, New Jersey, with her husband, Steve, daughter, Catherine, and newborn son, Joshua. She would like you to know that her photograph was taken during her second pregnancy—and that she really doesn't look this fat in real life.